NEW APPROACHES TO RELIGION AND POWER

Series editor: Joerg Rieger

While the relationship of religion and power is a perennial topic, it only continues to grow in importance and scope in our increasingly globalized and diverse world. Religion, on a global scale, has openly joined power struggles, often in support of the powers that be. But at the same time, religion has made major contributions to resistance movements. In this context, current methods in the study of religion and theology have created a deeper awareness of the issue of power: Critical theory, cultural studies, postcolonial theory, subaltern studies, feminist theory, critical race theory, and working class studies are contributing to a new quality of study in the field. This series is a place for both studies of particular problems in the relation of religion and power as well as for more general interpretations of this relation. It undergirds the growing recognition that religion can no longer be studied without the study of power.

Series editor:

Joerg Rieger is Wendland-Cook Professor of Constructive Theology in the Perkins School of Theology at Southern Methodist University.

Titles:

No Longer the Same: Religious Others and the Liberation of Christian Theology
David R. Brockman

The Subject, Capitalism, and Religion: Horizons of Hope in Complex Societies
Jung Mo Sung

Imaging Religion in Film: The Politics of Nostalgia
M. Gail Hamner

Spaces of Modern Theology: Geography and Power in Schleiermacher's World
Steven R. Jungkeit

Transcending Greedy Money: Interreligious Solidarity for Just Relations
Ulrich Duchrow and Franz J. Hinkelammert

Foucault, Douglass, Fanon, and Scotus in Dialogue: On Social Construction and Freedom
Cynthia R. Nielsen

Lenin, Religion, and Theology
Roland Boer

In Search of God's Power in Broken Bodies: A Theology of Maum
Hwa-Young Chong

The Reemergence of Liberation Theologies: Models for the Twenty-First Century
Edited by Thia Cooper

Theological Perspectives for Life, Liberty, and the Pursuit of Happiness: Public Intellectuals for the Twenty-First Century
Edited by Ada Maria Isasi-Diaz, Mary McClintock Fulkerson, and Rosemary Carbine

Religion, Theology, and Class
Edited by Joerg Rieger

Messianism Against Christology: Resistance Movements, Folk Arts, and Empire
James W. Perkinson

Decolonial Judaism: Triumphal Failures of Barbaric Thinking
Santiago Slabodsky

Trinitarian Theology and Power Relations: God Embodied
Meredith Minister

Pastoral Power Beyond Psychology's Marginalization: Resisting the Discourses of the Psy-Complex
Philip Browning Helsel

Pastoral Power Beyond Psychology's Marginalization
Resisting the Discourses of the Psy-Complex

Philip Browning Helsel

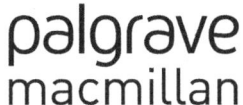

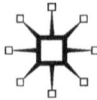

PASTORAL POWER BEYOND PSYCHOLOGY'S MARGINALIZATION
Copyright © Philip Browning Helsel, 2015.

All rights reserved.

First published in 2015 by
PALGRAVE MACMILLAN®
in the United States—a division of St. Martin's Press LLC,
175 Fifth Avenue, New York, NY 10010.

Where this book is distributed in the UK, Europe and the rest of the world, this is by Palgrave Macmillan, a division of Macmillan Publishers Limited, registered in England, company number 785998, of Houndmills, Basingstoke, Hampshire RG21 6XS.

Palgrave Macmillan is the global academic imprint of the above companies and has companies and representatives throughout the world.

Palgrave® and Macmillan® are registered trademarks in the United States, the United Kingdom, Europe and other countries.

ISBN: 978-1-137-49782-6

Library of Congress Cataloging-in-Publication Data

Helsel, Philip Browning.
  Pastoral power beyond psychology's marginalization : resisting the discourses of the psy-complex / Philip Browning Helsel.
      pages cm.—(New approaches to religion and power)
  Includes bibliographical references and index.
  ISBN 978-1-137-49782-6

  1. Pastoral counseling. 2. Poor—Mental health. 3. Working class—Mental health. 4. Poor—Mental health services. 5. Poor—Pastoral counseling. 6. Poverty—Psychological aspects. I. Title.
BV4012.2.H4254 2015
253.5—dc23   2015012948

A catalogue record of the book is available from the British Library.

Design by Newgen Knowledge Works (P) Ltd., Chennai, India.

First edition: October 2015

10 9 8 7 6 5 4 3 2 1

To Carolyn, for love and wisdom each step of the way

Contents

Acknowledgments	ix
Introduction	1
1 Social Class and Mental Illness in a Neoliberal Era	19
2 Psychiatric Power and the Limits of Biomedical Diagnosis	53
3 In Their Own Words: Mental Health Consumers, Survivors, and Ex-Patients	81
4 Pastoral Counseling and Social-Class Shame	121
5 The Counter-Conducts of Pastoral Power	155
6 An Integrative Vision for Pastoral Power	183
Notes	203
Bibliography	231
Index	247

Acknowledgments

This book has been written with the help of many thoughtful colleagues, friends, and students.

My primary word of gratitude is for all those c/s/x activists who shared their stories with me, starting from my first field education chaplaincy placement at Trenton Psychiatric Hospital and continuing into congregational ministry. Their honesty, courage, and willingness to let me be a partner to their stories has been a powerful experience.

I am also grateful to those scholars who encouraged me to consider economic issues specifically in my work. Ongoing conversations with Jeremy Posadas, Bruce Rogers-Vaughn, and Joerg Rieger have been especially helpful in this regard.

Generous scholars in the field have read drafts of this book, including the faculty at Boston College School of Theology and Ministry—from which I was granted writing leave—and Carolyn Browning Helsel, who read the entire manuscript. Likewise, I have benefited from the editorial assistance of Kevin Dowd, Ian Parelius, and Ryan Cosse. Friends such as David Cunnigham and Ben Broderick were helpful conversation partners.

I am grateful for my children Caleb and Evelyn who coped with the time I devoted to this project and shared their own publications with me. Their work is an inspiration to me.

As I worked on this book, I often thought of my peers in Anderson, Indiana, where I grew up, many of whom continue to endure the economic downturn and the traumas of living in a former factory town. Their stories impacted my thinking and writing: I am grateful for the ways that they struggle with and transform the world around them.

Introduction

During my seminary training I worked at one of the oldest psychiatric hospitals in the nation in an urban context and visited "chronic" patients who had been in the hospital for decades. Working at this large institution exposed me to the practice of confinement that is unique to mental hospitals. I noted the racial stratification of psychiatry, with white doctors organizing treatment and African Americans cleaning the rooms. I noticed how staff rarely talked to patients.

In a separate experience I worked at another psychiatric hospital/addiction treatment unit in a suburban context where patients stayed a few days or weeks. At this small institution, with more resources, the predominantly white staff seemed to offer in-depth education and therapeutic programming.

These two hospitals, about 17 miles apart, were two different worlds that resemble our divided nation. Indeed, in this book I argue that psychiatric treatment is one of the chief mirrors through which we can explore the true values of our times, namely, who is seen as worthy, who is understood, who is cherished, and who is abandoned. In these two different hospitals "patients" were being treated in different ways. Thus, mental illness becomes an interpretive frame through which to understand our society.[1] The difference in social setting and activities reflected important messages given about class, race, and identity in America.

This book is about the psychological impact of social class in an age of massive income inequity, rising unemployment, and soaring debt. Also, it is a book about how this psychological impact from the social world is inadequately interpreted when people are understood through an exclusively biomedical framework, as in much of modern American psychiatry. I argue that understanding the mental distress impact of the new economy can lead to greater solidarity with psychologically affected persons by redistributing necessary resources to them and also recognizing their voice. Redistribution is about making sure that persons have what is necessary to survive; recognition is about making sure their voices are heard.

Books about mental illness in pastoral care and counseling tend to favor the psychiatric frame, often accepting biomedical diagnostics without critiquing the power of psychiatry. Indeed, ministers and pastoral caregivers often feel ill-equipped to care for persons with mental difficulties so they refer them to other "experts" with similar class and educational backgrounds to themselves. Current approaches to mental illness in the pastoral counseling literature thus implicitly foster the diagnostic frame of psychiatry by reinforcing its categories, perhaps encouraging churches to be more hospitable to the mentally ill while leaving the framework of mental illness largely intact. At the same time, any redistribution that is offered by churches and ministers is often done under the rubric of charity, seen as a one-time gift for uplift. Since mental illness is often bound up with economic injustice, it is our responsibility to prevent it, and not just treat it.

I write as a white Presbyterian minister who teaches pastoral care at a Catholic school of theology. While growing up in Bangkok, Thailand, and then in Anderson, Indiana, I saw two sides of globalization in a neoliberal era. As an adolescent in Indiana, I saw my friends diagnosed with mental illness when their families were disintegrating. All around us rose the spectral ruins of automobile manufacturers, abandoned and covering the landscape in vast acres, a dystopic nightmare. Much of the social suffering I saw around me in the Rust Belt community where I was raised was related to vast unemployment and economic inequity. There was a palpable feeling of public despair, which was sometimes attributed to the psychologies of presumably mentally ill individuals. In my professional life as a board-certified chaplain in mental health institutions, counselor, and minister, I have been increasingly moved by the fact that we misinterpret much of the social suffering of our time with our given categories for mental illness. My own journey from working-class roots to professional identity has been a complex one. While now a beneficiary of middle class status and prestige, a privilege that comes through being an academic and a professional, I still sometimes feel estranged from both the middle class and my working-class roots.[2] These are the issues that undergird the book, whose argument attempts to address the economic suffering that underlies this despair in a complex fashion, interpreting the distress not as a sign of something unbalanced in one's brain, rooted in one's genes, but rather rooted in the stress and trauma of working-class experience.

Social Class and Mental Distress

An exclusively biomedical approach to mental illness is missing something significant since much of what people are suffering from today could be described as economic oppression. Today people are working in worse conditions than ever before, often with less pay and fewer rights. They face frequent unemployment and carry heavy debts simply to survive. All of these factors have direct psychological effects that are not described clearly by dominant medical frameworks for mental illness.

Emerging research indicates that class dynamics directly contributes to mental distress. Mounting evidence shows links between mental turmoil and one's position in a less-privileged social class.[3] Persons in working-class positions are more likely to experience mental distress than managers, as are persons who feel that their labor has been exploited.[4] Some of the most pressing effects of the current economic crisis—income inequity, unemployment, debt, and home foreclosure—have distinctive impacts on psychological well-being.

Research suggests that persons who own a home or a car are less likely to experience mental distress, while chronic unemployment is a leading cause for suicide.[5] Studies have even demonstrated how impoverishment impacts persons in childhood, producing stress that influences early childhood development and leads to anxiety and depression in adolescence.[6] Since biomedical models of mental illness systematically exclude all but the most general economic information, these links between economic factors and mental suffering are not theorized effectively.

The paradox is that an exclusively biomedical model of mental illness obscures from us the distinctive causes and sources of suffering that stem from these new economic times. The changes that we have seen in our society in the last 20 to 30 years can be described as neoliberalism, which David Harvey defined as

> a theory of political and economic practices that proposes that human well being can best be advanced by liberating individual entrepreneurial freedoms and skills within an institutional framework characterized by strong private property rights, free markets, and free trade.[7]

It is important to note that neoliberalism is not simply an economic system; it is also a culture that promotes a certain view of the person.[8] A distinctive aspect of this culture is its tendency to place internal blame for suffering that is rooted in the social realm. At the same time, there is the implicit expectation that everyone should be able to succeed.

As the market increasingly comes to define various aspects of persons' lives,[9] neoliberalism silences organizing and labor movements, as well as movements for self-definition and intersectional rights.[10]

For example, major depression first entered the diagnostic manuals in 1980, just when neoliberal governments told us "there is no society, only individuals [and their families]."[11] Bruce Rogers-Vaughn argues that biomedical psychiatry, which broadened the mental illness framework at the same time that it individualized the consumer of mental health, has turned suffering into a market and thus created a culture. This culture has been fostered by direct-to-consumer advertising that has promoted an individualized view of mental distress that is simply meant to be overcome.

Rogers-Vaughn carefully nuances his point, stating that depression is a complex phenomenon, and argues that an exclusively biomedical view of depression as rooted in the brain or the genes obscures the fact that, with rising economic inequity, depression should be considered, in the words of Ann Cvetcovitch, a "public feeling."[12] If a greater number of people sense that they do not quite measure up and that they may be failures in an economic world intent on cutthroat competition, and if more opportunities are available to see their suffering as being treatable by medication only, then we are obviously missing much of the tenor of our emotional times. Rather than silencing the voice of depression, Rogers-Vaughn argues that we must listen to it, noting how it reflects on our wider society.

Rogers-Vaughn makes a compelling case that mood disorders are more prevalent in societies with a great deal of inequality. Neoliberalism seeks to maximize profits, and in the process incites persons to measure themselves primarily in economic terms. He argues that depression in persons is a response to the message that their monetary value is the only meaning placed on their lives.[13] He interprets the rise in antidepressant medication as a stifling of the potential for political resistance against the imposition of an unjust system.[14]

What we have on our hands is widespread confusion about what ails us and what we should do about it. Indeed, there seem to be a range of professionals in a variety of disciplines who are happy to individualize a person's mental suffering as a disease and chart its course, applying medicine to the problem. By contrast we need to find ways of listening to the distinctive suffering of our times and enabling persons to respond directly to what causes that suffering.

In this book I argue that social class is an important way to understand the suffering of neoliberalism. On one hand, social class could just refer to the fact that these changes under neoliberalism were made by persons who were elite and who fostered their own interest by moving companies abroad, eviscerating unions, and keeping wages low. On the other hand, social class is a more complex phenomenon since it involves the relationship between workers and employers. For this book, social class means not simply "collections of families and individuals who have similar levels of, and access to, scarce and valued resources over time"[15] but also *the interdependent antagonism that links workers and owners together over time as owners exploit the surplus labor of workers primarily to further capitalist profit and thereby forcefully exclude many seeming nonproducers.* Note that this definition—which I explore further in chapter 1—includes relationships of production and talks about the core conditions of capitalism. Unfortunately, many of our current ways of describing and managing psychological distress do not grapple with the concrete realities of social class.

The Psy-Complex

Nikolas Rose coined the term the "psy-complex" in his discussion of the development of psychological testing in the United Kingdom during World War I, and his definition indicated that it included various disciplines of psychiatry, psychology, and social work, as well as the institutional settings in which they are deployed.[16] Drawing heavily from Michel Foucault, he argued that the psy-complex helped persons describe various aspects of their lives under the rubric of an overarching theme and that this contributed to the production of a certain kind of identity, an identity as a *psyche*. In this book, I address how the system of mental health diagnosis and treatment exerts a social control over persons that obscures some significant aspects of their suffering.

In chapter 2, I state that the psy-complex includes the tendency to posit internal structures of thought or mind to interpret factors that are inherently social. It often includes a kind of "methodological individualism" along with a preference for organic medical explanations of mental health rooted in the brain or genes of an individual. Persons who work in the psy-complex are, by virtue of their training, often middle class or upper class, although their own class position rarely enters into their official judgments.

Rose emphasizes that the psy-complex constitutes the collaboration of official human sciences with technologies of control and normalization. He did not adequately describe what this control or normalization might be for, or what use it served in society.

What purpose does the psy-complex play in the twenty-first century? It offers metaphors that structure a person in individualistic terms, with mental health or illness located squarely within their own brain or genes. This individualizing tendency does not adequately attend to social explanations for suffering, such as those drawn from social psychiatry and mental health epidemiology, that look at how economic, racial, and gender oppression interact with mental illness. Even when the psy-complex may attend to some contextual factors, it tends to do so as "risk factors" incidental to a larger pathology. The psy-complex is both reified and supported by training schools and official credentials, and it is supplemented by major federal grants that are interested in organic causes of mental illness but not social and environmental stressors.

People who are seen as poor are often diagnosed with a mental illness.[17] Given the rise in the neoliberal perspective in which capital accumulation is highly valued over other social goods, working-class communities become sites of state-based interventions. For instance, social workers and other professionals within the psy-complex intervene in the lives of working-class persons to determine whether they are still eligible for government aid.[18] In this sense, persons who work hard to survive every day are more heavily managed by the language and practices of the psy-complex. At a wealthy private psychiatric hospital, case files for persons covered by Medicaid were bulging with reports, while private-pay patients had only a few documents in their files.[19]

The language of psychiatry and psychology, when applied to the conditions of poverty, can implicitly naturalize poverty by making it seem as if the poor person is responsible for a problem existing inside him or herself or within his or her community. The "culture of poverty" discourse describes poor persons as "unwilling or unable to respond appropriately to the values, rewards, and expectations that formed the... larger society."[20] This kind of discourse lays primary blame for poverty on working-class persons, thus contributing to their stigmatization while obscuring structural changes that have led to more widespread poverty for many. Here is an example of what can happen when being in the working class becomes the object of the psy-complex discourse: if poverty universally has these effects on people, and if they need expert help to "break out of" its cycles, then poverty again becomes the responsibility of the individual rather than the result of structural injustices perpetuated by vested interests. Impoverished persons are often described as implicitly "dangerous" or delinquent and needing correction.[21]

Once people are perceived as poor, they enter into the psy-complex as subjects to be managed. This transformation of discourse offers an internalized interpretation of their economic suffering, when in fact social causes have contributed to their distress. Economic realities are increasingly being represented in medical terms through biological and psychological models that do not account for the role that working-class experience plays in our understanding of health. In my description of the two psychiatric hospitals at the beginning, one of the most startling facts was the radically different economic condition at each hospital. Among the most problematic effects of psy-complex discourse *about* poverty is that it implicitly blames impoverished persons and their communities for effects that are structural and even global, thus reinforcing a sense of interiority and shame when political resistance would be a more appropriate response.

Persons who work in the psy-complex are often responsible for identifying problems within persons and ameliorating them. They are involved in a system in which social control is often exerted through psychological medicine. Yet they are also able to resist social control, as when a social worker challenged her supervisor's diagnosis in a case conference meeting,[22] or when a counselor in a welfare office worked with clients to make sure that they could get the maximum benefits.[23] The psy-complex tends to focus on individuals and their families rather than social factors, positing an "ideal" world of thoughts and motivations whereas the horizon of corporate, media, and global factors is actually even more significant than one's own thoughts, cognitions, and family relationship in influencing one's behavior.[24]

The psy-complex is the conceptual category that emphasizes biomedicalization of distress in ever-widening variations, such as the pathologization of grief at the loss of a loved one.[25] The psy-complex is reinforced by daily television advertisements that promise happiness through psychotropic medications and also by the massive corporate infiltration of psychiatry by pharmaceutical companies who run the agenda for the mental health industry.[26] The difficulty with the psy-complex is that if it defines a person's suffering as primarily originating from their own personality, body chemistry, or family, it underestimates the complex and interconnected levels of oppression inherent in modern-day neoliberalism by positing individual blame for social problems.

Psychology's Marginalization

On the opposite end of the psy-complex's social control is a positive and helpful version of psychology, one that attends to subjective interpersonal experience such as the attempts to survive chronic and debilitating conditions. This kind of *psychology that counts* attends to factors such as work, money, gender, race, privilege, and personal as well as structural feelings that interpret these realities. This psychology would have little to do with illness or treatment and would not be a scientific psychology based on a pragmatic cure for behavior, but would attend to the subjective experience of what it feels like to live in a neoliberal era.

David Smail offers one such reframing of psychology. He notes, "It's hard to see how I can avoid 'psychology' at least as *part* of my enterprise," but he insists that his version of the discipline is as much concerned about what goes on in the world as it is with what goes on in a persons head.[27] He clarifies his project as aimed at what it means to experience "avoidable" human suffering in our bodies and selves, and he suggests that psychology should give us tools to understand and respond to this suffering.[28] Critiquing a psy-complex notion of the importance of an individual's thoughts or intentions, he argues that most psychology focuses persons on an inner world that does not go beyond what is inside their own skulls.[29] Likewise, it makes a similar error of focusing treatment on what is proximal to that person—their own family and kin-network—rather than focusing on influential outside power structures. By contrast, Smail argues for what he calls a "social environmentalist psychology," which, rather than helping the person in their own thoughts discover insight into their behaviors, would "help the person achieve 'outsight,' such that the causes of distress can be demystified and the extent of their own responsibility for their condition put into its proper perspective."[30]

Psychology should help us map the widespread emotional distress of our times, as Ann Cvetkovich has done in her work on depression. She argues that depression is a "public feeling" related as much to political events as interpersonal ones.[31] Maintaining that we must find ways to bring feelings back into politics and bring the political into our discussion of feelings, she indicates that this could mean hearing widespread national and chronic trauma such as racial oppression, class suffering, and the marginalization of various sexual identities through the lens of a revitalized psychology.

Additionally, we must find ways of talking about what is painful and shameful. Voicing marginalized experiences allow these silenced themes to emerge. In her book *Where We Stand: Class Matters*, bell hooks describes how her own family of origin never talked about money.[32] When her family moved into a middle-class neighborhood, a kind of pride kept her mother from being too glad about leaving the other past behind. Likewise, when hooks wanted to go to an expensive out-of-state college, her desire was named "sin" rather than class transgression.[33] The primary dynamic that hooks describes in talking about class is "shame." She notes, "When I went to fancy colleges where money and status defined one's place in the scheme of things, I found myself an object of curiosity, ridicule, and even contempt from my classmates because of my class background. At times I felt shame."[34] Rogers-Vaughn suggests that greater inequality leads to greater shame, as persons engage in shame-based expenditure cascades in which they shop as a way of shoring up their image of themselves.[35]

Without addressing the central role that shame plays in many of our social encounters, it is difficult to address why consumer culture is such a powerful influence on US society. Persons who are influenced by class shame are impacted by the feelings of emptiness and need. In a world in which people bombarded by images of very wealthy individuals and their consumptive patterns, a kind of chronic shame and rage set in for persons who are excluded from this wealth and seemingly unable to "make ends meet."

Addressing painful and unspoken realities that surround social class is one important step in changing the systems in which we unconsciously operate. To do this means that we plumb the best of our traditions and also critique them. On the one hand, this kind of psychology could be used, as in the work of early social psychology pioneers such as Harry Stack Sullivan as described by Philip Cushman, to "identify and ameliorate the 'root causes' of poverty, racism" and other oppressions.[36] In order to do this, Sullivan suggested, we must challenge universal ahistoricism in our disciplines along with its "unanalyzed class bias."[37]

I argue that psychology involves attention to subjective interpersonal experience, especially that of unnecessary suffering, and that it also highlights persons' attempts to cope with and survive chronic and debilitating conditions. With careful attention to the biomedicalization of everyday experience, such as people's tendency to describe themselves as a "risk" or "liability," this kind of psychology attends to the suffering of the perceived failure to be a neoliberal subject, and the uncomfortable feelings that can attend such experience, such as shame and personal failing.

Rather than positing elaborate inner conceptions of selfhood to respond to social suffering, this approach turns to the world outside with political feelings, challenging the divisions between public and private and the exclusion of emotions from the public sphere.[38] The critique of the psy-complex rested on its methodological individualism. This kind of psychology, by contrast, approaches public realities with personal feelings and addresses these feelings directly in a public venue.

Psychology's marginalization has happened through market-based models of mind and body that tend to reduce people to certain quantifiable factors. Recovering psychology from its marginalization means taking account of the social environmental psychology that comes from living in a neoliberal age, often psychically "well beyond our means," and grappling with this in a public fashion.[39] Bringing hidden feelings of shame, rage, and powerlessness to bear on circumstances of mass oppression involves revealing the pain that has come from decades of marginalization and despair.

As I argued previously, this book is about the psychological impact of social class in an age of massive income inequity, rising unemployment, and soaring debt. Also, it is a book about how this psychological impact from the social world is marginalized when persons are understood through an exclusively biomedical framework, as in modern American psychiatry.

Too little attention has been focused in pastoral care and counseling on the conditions in which people have to work and how these conditions contribute to their social suffering. Researchers have discovered that a lack of money does produce unhappiness, but an excess of it does not contribute to happiness at all.[40] A focus on money, investments, and social inequity shows how people are increasingly invited to measure themselves on the basis of capital rather than meaning making, leading to an elision of significance for many persons who measure themselves based on money alone rather than social relationships, community, neighborhood, or other supports. Indeed, other sources, such as theological anthropology and reflections on the importance of work must be used to supplement our pastoral theology at this point, because our reflections on social class seem to be absent and our analysis of mental illness lacks a rigorous exploration of the economic impact on emotional distress.

On one hand, this book is about economic inequity and its psychological effects: it is fundamentally an argument for more just redistribution (the redistributive pole), which is economic restructuring to reduce differences in income and wealth that are unjust.[41] Redistribution refers not only to income, but also to how wealth transfers across the generations. My argument in this book is that the redistribution pole has been weakly theorized in academic life and in my discipline of pastoral care and counseling specifically. Understanding the psychological impact of social class means directly addressing the subordination of workers and those excluded from the economy through redistribution.

At the same time, dealing with this kind of suffering often involves a struggle for recognition (the recognition pole) and the effort to create a world in which different types people would not be stigmatized and would have a chance to fully participate in society. In writing this book I have discussed that it is seldom possible to write about social class without also writing about race, but I have also found that it is impossible to understand class strictly in terms of an analysis of race. Dealing with the problems of economics often engages with the politics of identity—are the "poor" a particular kind of people with their own identity? Understanding the identity politics of the new economy means grappling with how the marginalization of the poor includes stereotypes about them.[42] As Nancy Fraser has argued, many struggles for justice involve both the pole of redistribution and recognition, and throughout this book we keep both in view.[43]

In this book I argue that the biomedicalization of psychiatry keeps us from seeing a crucial factor at play in the new economy—how many people are suffering mental distress as a result of income inequity, lack of proper housing, despair from the lack of hope, and other economic factors (the redistributive pole). The issue of mental illness is, in our times, frequently an issue of proper redistribution, since much mental and emotional suffering could be prevented through social class change. There are cases in which economic factors do not play a role but these are few.[44]

Nevertheless, once people come into contact with the mental health system, they often come away with a new identity label drawn from psychiatric nosology to describe their symptoms (the recognition pole). They sometimes join a new social category as a person who has been psychiatrized. In this condition, people sometimes band together to collectively name their own experience over-against an expert definition. Some of the research in this book is dedicated to exploring the recognition pole of psychiatric survivor movements and how these movements intersect with social class. Yet even these recognition movements require advocacy on the redistribution pole, since mental distress frequently leads to homelessness and lack of social support.

Disability and Mental Health

In the United States we are not very tolerant of different behaviors. We tend to medicalize and pathologize difference, hoping that persons who exhibit differences will go away. Indeed, we reward psychologists and psychiatrists who are able to *name* difference by linking it to an internal life. It is altogether too easy then, once someone has a different name attached to him or her, to render that person invisible by placing them in a community without mental and emotional supports. Indeed, it seems natural in our time to do so.

Yet all of us are potentially different. In the 1980s differently abled rights activists coined the term "temporarily able bodied" to describe the experience of those deemed to not have a disability.[45] Likewise, we might say that many of us are "temporarily sane."[46]

Taking this perspective would mean that we value the concerns of persons diagnosed with mental illness as our own, joining in a form of active solidarity with them. In order for this solidarity to be effective, it is necessary to hear their concerns from their own viewpoint rather than from an outsider's "expert" perspective. Solidarity is possible only through sustained attention to another's voice, to how they name and define their own experience, and ultimately to how they create conscious communities around these stories.[47] There are a range of forces that impact the lives of persons who have a mental health diagnosis—the stunning multiplicity of these factors can be overwhelming—from unemployment to chronic pain; and from disrupted family relationships to limited options for fulfilling work. Especially given the widespread economic downturn, the lack of proper social safety nets, and the psychological effects of these changes, achieving solidarity with persons who have had mental illness also means advocating for economic solidarity.

Sometimes a person is considered a problem because they are of a different gender, race, class, or sexual orientation than the person in power in a given situation. At other times a person is described as being a problem when that person is poor. Even one who talks differently or walks differently than others is sometimes considered a problem. What I have found in this research is that a person who is perceived as different is more likely to be diagnosed as mentally ill and this diagnosis can make others take that person less seriously, leading to a potential diminishment of the person's rights.

Through these pages I hope that you can imagine what it would be like to be diagnosed with a mental illness because of economic stress and how you might respond to the experience, especially if you sensed that the daily stress and pressures of making ends meet had lead to a mental health diagnosis. Named by others with a category, measured by a battery of tests, put through any number of therapeutic techniques, persons can become fatigued from or frightened by their encounters with these systems-that-treat-symptoms. When these forms of difference can be thought of as "symptoms," symptomatology can overshadow everyday life. People seek to be known and heard as more than simply an object to be acted upon to remove symptoms.

C/S/X Activism

Since the 1960s and 1970s persons diagnosed with mental illness have begun organizing so that their own perspective could be heard and so that they could negotiate with psychiatric power. Early efforts, deemed "anti-psychiatry" by its detractors, stated that mental health users needed to be able to define their own realities rather than having a name imposed on them. The movement has advocated for a range of rights in relation to the experience of being diagnosed with mental illness, from informed consent—including discussion of the side effects of psychiatric medication—to psychiatric advanced directives in which certain treatments could be refused. At the same time, some activists have organized against involuntary commitment.[48] Chapter 3 turns to consumer/survivor/ex-patient (hereafter c/s/x) narratives to see how these narratives challenge the social and economic structures of our time.

On one end of the movement are "consumers" who may accept the epistemological categories of mental illness while advocating for greater rights within the system. On the other end are "survivors" who describe "treatment" methods as being torture and advocate for the end of psychiatry.[49] "Ex-patients" criticize the permanent status of being labeled as mentally ill. C/s/x groups offer peer support that critiques how social power is used in psychiatric practice from an insider perspective, often using first-person language rather than third-person clinical terminology. This line of critique is quite different from a stigma-busting emphasis, which can be accomplished while holding in place psychiatry's capacity to classify experience.[50]

In order to understand the importance of psychiatric power and its links to pastoral care and counseling, we must attend to the voices of those most impacted by a biomedical model of mental illness. There has been an important trend toward analyzing the impact of economic factors in these groups, especially those who have critiqued institutionalization in favor of jobs and housing. C/s/x narratives often lead to practical considerations, such as good employment and lodging, freedom from harassment, exemption from criminalization in the penal system, as well as the voice necessary for self-determination, and these are all significant avenues of activism. Rather than seeing c/s/x communities as objects which society must act upon, this approach sees these communities' concerns as a prism through which to take stock of modern US society, especially the fact that many persons are still isolated from others and subjected to cruel and degrading practices because of their presumed difference. In a religious sense, hearing the communal stories of c/s/x activists makes one a "partner" who has ethical responsibilities rather than a mere spectator.[51]

At the same time, a national study suggests that class and economic analysis may still be a very important and undertheorized aspect of c/s/x activism.[52] In examining the benefits of c/s/x organizing efforts, a group of researchers and c/s/x activists found that net income was the only social position factor that made a difference in whether people could benefit from c/s/x organizing.[53] This indicates that c/s/x activism must be integrated with broader movements for economic justice since the achievement of rights in this arena is closely connected to economic goals such as earning just wages, having appropriate chances in one's life, or work that is free from exploitation.[54]

Pastoral Power

Ministers are often sought out to make sense of mental suffering by persons in their communities and are thus front-line responders to emotional distress so prevalent in a neoliberal era. I describe the ability to interpret suffering as a form of power, and religious leaders in communities have *pastoral power* regardless of whether they are officially ordained. Michel Foucault used the term *pastoral power* to describe the clergy's responsibility.[55] I use the term more broadly to indicate the symbolic religious power that is used to help persons understand and interpret their faith in relationship to their life circumstances. Ministers could be chaplains (hospital, psychiatric, or military), church educators, congregational and parish clergy, pastoral counselors, religion teachers, or campus ministers.

Pastoral power refers to the ability to help people interpret their lives that is conferred through the interplay of three sources. These sources include the establishment of trust (which is accumulated from the amount of time a minister has travelled with another and the extent of the invitation extended to help them make sense of their suffering); the symbolic authority accorded to the minister (which refers to the official religious power given through the ordained status or license, indicating the combination of professional licensure, education, and religious symbolism granted with a particular community's meaning-making system); and intercultural status (which is the extent to which one shares culture, gender, sexual orientation, national identity, extent of physical disability, age position, and the extent to which this helps build a bridge of shared understanding through similarity). Once these three factors intersect, a person has pastoral power in a situation that includes the ability to help persons name and interpret their suffering. Although pastoral power is the site of the misuse of power it is also potentially the site of resistance against various forms of reductionism and social control.

Understanding social class is essential to the proper exercise of pastoral power in the twenty-first century. There is an unprecedented extent of economic suffering in people's communities today and ministers are often first responders in a variety of psychiatric and psychological events that follow from this distress. A congregant attempts to take her life after a period of unemployment; another enters into despair after he is removed from his rental property. This leads to his hospitalization in a psychiatric hospital. In these circumstances, ministers engage in a variety of forms of interpretation of suffering. Some of these interpretations may be drawn from the language of faith and prayer and others may be drawn from an exclusively biomedical model of mental illness.

Structure of the Book

In chapter 1, I explore the nature and extent of economic suffering and argue that this suffering impacts the emotional lives of persons, contributing to what are described as mental illnesses. In this chapter I describe massive changes that have occurred to the economy under neoliberalism in the last 30 years and explore the psychic effects on persons impacted by unemployment and debt. This chapter shows how neoliberalism is actually the effect of social class, and describes how understanding of social class as a relationship can lead to shared solidarity between persons in working-class positions.

In chapter 2 I explain the psy-complex biomedical model of mental illness and historicize it as a development in modern neoliberalism. An exclusively biomedical concept of mental illness reduces psychic suffering to brain diseases and searches for an organic basis for the illness. I describe the rise of psychopharmacology as a corporate practice that has reinforced descriptive psychiatry. Relativizing psychiatric discourse as a context-specific practice with sweeping power implications, this chapter shows how psychiatric discourse becomes a way of labeling persons from particular classes, genders, and races, and how this often occurs as a way of managing the poor, reifying them as an identity, and treating them as a sick subgroup. Exploring deinstitutionalization, transinstitutionalization—moving persons out of mental hospitals and into prisons—and the rise of managed care, this chapter explains the crisis of emotional suffering in an era when everyone is expected to be responsible for themselves.

In chapter 3 I analyze counter-voices that challenge the psy-complex's exclusive reliance on a biomedical model. Since the voices of persons affected by psychiatric power are rarely included in the official discourse of the psy-complex, I focus on group discussions of c/s/x activists who deploy the language of rights to critique the psychiatric frame, insisting on their capacity to name their own experience and locate these discussions in an intersectional analysis. Exploring the narratives of c/s/x communities as having overlapping concerns for both recognition and also redistribution, this chapter looks at the importance of *intersectionality*, how being diagnosed as mentally ill can interact with other forms of oppression such as belonging to the working class or to a racial or ethnic group that has been marginalized. Understanding the intersecting nature of oppressions is only possible when the redistributive pole is kept in the forefront. This chapter explores how social class intersects with a variety of rights-based issues in c/s/x activism, such as forced hospitalization and/or medication, psychiatric advanced directives, shock treatments (ECT) and other human rights concerns.

In chapter 4 I explore the practice of pastoral counseling as a potential site of resistance. Although pastoral counselors are frequently responsible for psychiatric diagnoses and thus share the power of the clinical frame, they are also capable, through a psychology that engages the entire social environment, of attending to the oppressions of social class. I operationalize Wright's notion of social class as a relationship into a series of pastoral counseling inquiries. The particular goal of this exploration is to reduce the potential shame of being in a working-class position and foster a sense of solidarity. This requires a redefining of the practice of counseling, away from idealistic models that emphasize the mind and cognitions or interpersonal family relationships. Instead, the counselor becomes a social-class advocate by examining their own class position and engaging in macro-level advocacy even while doing the micro-work of pastoral counseling.

In chapter 5, I explain the notion of pastoral power (shared trust, symbolic authority, and cultural similarity/difference) as it relates to broader ministry. In this chapter I explain Foucault's idea of the counter-conducts of pastoral power, namely *mysticism, community, asceticism, scripture,* and *eschatology,* as being border practices within Christianity.

In my distinctive take on the counter-conducts, I argue that they make this power available directly to the community as a source of authority and site of transformation.

In chapter 6 I make a claim that the perspectives of those who have suffered from pastoral power must transform religious communities. This chapter sets forth an integrative proposal that links the oppression of social identity with a practical argument for the transformation of religious communities around c/s/x concerns. This does not mean simply bringing the message of working-class activists to religious communities but rather understanding how the churches themselves can organize around the contextual oppressions that are involved in mental illness and working-class identities.

This book is about the kinds of *power* that ministers have to name another's suffering and how this power exists in a continuum with the psychiatric power to diagnose, treat, and administer medication. It links heretofore separated fields of discourse: economic analysis, social critical theory, and pastoral care, in order to show how pastoral care and counseling is itself a form of power. The goal is to craft more strategic practices that can foster the opportunity for voice and agency among those working-class persons effected by the practices of psychiatry and pastoral care.

There are several results that I hope come from this book. First, I believe that deconstructing the psy-complex in this manner should lead to engaged community action around a range of intersectional rights, including economic, gender, racial, ethnic, and differently abled activism. The priority remains on economic justice since it appears that this is crucial in c/s/x activism and since this focus has the ability to mobilize across differences.[56] In this approach, ministers and pastoral counselors will still do their ministry work of counseling but will link it more closely to political action, advocacy, and community organizing. In order to engage in this activism, ministers need to understand the pervasiveness of economic suffering and how it has shaped the climate in which so many are diagnosed with mental illness. They also need to use their authority to create communities of resistance in which people can organize greater rights and access to limited goods, as well as greater capacity for self-determination.

CHAPTER 1

Social Class and Mental Illness in a Neoliberal Era

In the Frontline documentary film, interviewer Bill Moyers chronicles the lives of *Two American Families* over a span of two decades in Milwaukee, WI, to explore the impact of the closing of factories and the rise of a low-wage service sector economy.[1] One family, the Stanleys, are African American and each parent had jobs at Briggs and Stratton before the factory closed. Once the factory closed, the father took a seven-dollar-an-hour job finishing basements while the mother worked in real estate. They experimented with opening their own business but had to close it because of a lack of interest. Throughout the film, Moyers expertly narrates the rising income inequity, the dissolution of jobs with living-wage pay and benefits, and the social impact on these families' lives. He notes that all these changes occurred during times of unprecedented growth in the Gross Domestic Product (GDP).

When he returns a decade later to interview the family in 2013, the mother, Jackie Stanley, nearly refuses to be interviewed by Moyers again, stating, "I thought I was a failure. I knew you thought I was a failure 'cause I didn't do it. We went backwards." Due to health problems, she quit her real estate job. Her business came to nothing. She concluded that she had not done enough to make it happen. "I really was ashamed," she told Moyers.[2]

In the twenty-first century we live in times of tremendous economic resources in the United States, even when rising inequity makes it impossible for people to make ends meet.[3] Because there is such an accent on personal initiative, people are likely to blame themselves for their suffering, just as Jackie Stanley did. In these times of crisis, pastoral care and counseling needs to interpret the context of economic suffering so that people can resist the shame of feeling personally responsible for economic suffering. Putting the blame in the right place, means understanding a class struggle that has redistributed income to the top one percent.[4]

The hypothesis of this chapter is that *much of the psychic suffering that people face in the new economy is preventable* because it has to do with unfair wages and a lack of decision-making power. Social class is more than just poverty research—it is about the conditions of workers— thus researching how social classes are *in relationship with one another* restores power back to workers. In order to understand this argument, readers need to challenge common stereotypes about the working class, such as the notion that they have individual traits that make them poor. Greater social responsibility is the goal of such research. In the current economic climate we can do a great deal of good, and avoid unnecessary suffering, by placing the conditions of work and income inequity at the foreground in pastoral theology.

Some use the notion of globalization to indicate that working-class rights are no longer an issue. If all the manufacturing jobs have gone overseas there is no grounds for working-class struggle.[5] This may seem to be the case in a global economy in which, through massive outsourcing of manufacturing, the new working class is now global.[6] Yet labor movements continue to win concessions in pay and working conditions. Fostering such movements is crucial to pastoral theology's approach to mental illness and emotional suffering in the twenty-first century.

If we do not accept this thesis, we misunderstand much distress by transposing it into personal psychic factors, and thinking that if we could only address these factors, people would become healthier. It is important that we understand the significance of money, how crucial people's income and wealth are to their psychic lives, and the ways in which they struggle because of the conditions of their work. Faced with increasing economic pressure, people are constructed, in the neoliberal economy described in the introduction, in terms of whether capital can flow freely through them.[7] If it cannot they are "deficient" and represent a "risk" to be managed and may describe themselves as "liabilities." On the other hand, if they can monetize themselves, they are seen as having "resources" and even "strengths."[8] People are described in the monetary terms of "risk" as "at-risk" teenagers. Social conditions are described through the language "risk factors." Unbridled accumulation of capital has become one of the most important goals of our times and thus it contributes to how persons describe themselves.[9] Even though the social factors arrayed against Mrs. Stanley were immense, she blamed herself for not succeeding in her business and described herself as failing. Ministers and pastoral counselors need to reject these individualistic attributions and replace them with critical tools that can help them evaluate the concept of social class.

Economic Conditions and Mental Illness

Much of the psychic suffering that we face as a society is preventable because it is shaped by economic conditions. In one of the largest studies of mental illness in the United States, almost all mental disorders were much higher among those with less education and lower income.[10] In this section I explore the extent to which mental illness is caused by economic stress. A meta-analysis of the relationship between socioeconomic factors and mental disorders concluded that 9 out of 12 major studies indicated an area's lower socioeconomic position or greater inequality was associated with mental disorder.[11]

Research has measured *material* concerns such as whether one owns a home or car and *psychosocial* concerns like job autonomy. While both kinds of measures are important, this section focuses primarily on material measures. In a large-scale study of depression, it was found that those with low educational attainment or low income are more likely to be diagnosed with depression, and people with incomes below $20,000 a year were twice as likely to be depressed as those with incomes of $70,000 a year.[12] In a long-term study that used psychiatric interviews, a supposedly more reliable measure than self-report, it was found that poverty increased the risk of depression two and a half times.[13] In terms of occupational social class, household service workers had three times the rate of depression as executives and these were reported at similar levels after a year's time. Being born to parents who were manual laborers made women twice as likely to be depressed and men four times as likely to be depressed, whereas having one parent who was middle class was a protective factor for depression.[14]

Material means are important even in cases of intersectional oppression. For example, in research among gay Latino men in New York and Miami, the influence of poverty was an important source of stress along with homophobia and racism.[15] Despite high levels of education, more than a quarter of these men were unemployed and many had recently looked for work. Financial hardship was a significant cause of stress for them and this effect could be seen independently of other variables. In the United States, there seems to be a two-to-three times higher prevalence for mood and substance abuse disorders and a four-fold higher prevalence overseas among working-class persons.[16]

Material measures have been important in the United Kingdom, where researchers measured what they called "standard of living," an aggregate of housing conditions (structural problems), the ability to save, the ownership of a house or car, and household income, and the researchers found that these factors were independently associated with mental illness "after adjusting for age, sex, social class, ethnicity" and a number of other factors.[17] Indeed, the findings were so compelling that the researchers suggested that standard of living factors accounted for "nearly one quarter of all cases" of mental illness after adjusting for other forms of potential marginalization, such as gender and ethnicity.[18]

In the case of depression, persons from a lower socioeconomic status were 1.8 times more likely than the wealthy to become depressed and experience persistent depression.[19] They found that low socioeconomic status was associated with panic, all types of phobias, and generalized anxiety, though the research was less clear about obsessive-compulsive disorder.[20]

While readers might have expected correlation among anxiety, depression, and socioeconomic status, even more seemingly "severe" mental illnesses such as schizophrenia have been linked to socioeconomic status. A study that indicated that as many as 19 years before treatment, those who later developed schizophrenia had a lower socioeconomic status.[21] There is a significant genetic component to a disease such as schizophrenia, but economic stress is also a contributing factor to whether or not people will develop the illness.[22]

Working-class people may also be exposed to conditions that lead to stress and mental illness. A foundational study explored the impact of being working class on persons who would eventually be diagnosed with schizophrenia. Being working class meant persons worked amidst more "noisome" occupations, including "excessive noise, hazardous conditions, extreme heat, extreme cold, excessive humidity, and aversive atmospheric conditions," and these occupations were in turn risk factors for schizophrenia.[23] This is especially important because of the age of onset of schizophrenia—often just as people are entering their first jobs. The authors of the study thereby argued that it was not "pre-existing vulnerability" but rather socioeconomic status that placed persons at risk for schizophrenia, especially the traumatic and stressful conditions of their first jobs.[24]

Economic suffering is a causal element in much, although not all, psychic suffering. Little wonder that Mrs. Stanley felt such personal distress. This is especially the case since the Great Recession, in which many more persons have been faced with unemployment, debt, and home foreclosure. The research presented here, undertaken before the recession, indicates that material measures such as income and possessions are a significant factor in the onset of many psychiatric disorders. In what follows, I trace the life-or-death psychic impact of the recent economic recession, offering an image of the suffering that is occurring in so many of our communities today.

Unemployment

The Great Recession of 2008 saw more than a doubling of unemployment, from four percent to ten percent. In the third quarter of 2010 two hundred million people worldwide were unemployed, and this was up a full third from 2008.[25] In the years since, the employment rate has fallen somewhat, but many are still underemployed.[26] Although some sectors of the economy have been growing, the long-term unemployed, nearly a third of all unemployed, has remained stable at 2.8 million.[27] This is a widespread problem.

It is clear that unemployment has a direct effect on psychological health that cannot be reduced to other factors. Persons who were unemployed were more than twice as likely to have psychological problems as the employed.[28] In one study that analyzed factory closures, they found that it was the situation of unemployment, rather than previous mental distress, that led directly to suffering, thus disproving the hypothesis that unemployment only affects those who had previous mental health problems.[29] People who live in countries with weak employment protections suffered more than those who were in countries that regulated how employees could be fired.[30]

Being unemployed often lead to a paradoxical situation—people were deprived of the very resources that would help them to get emotional support and practical help during the difficult time of job loss. People who are unemployed have more difficulty finding health care or psychological help;[31] they also tend to blame themselves for their job loss,[32] sometimes leading to what has been called a "chain of adversity."[33] Persons who are unemployed have less social contacts—a direct contributor to mental distress,[34] and also report less self-continuity across time.[35] People with preexisting medical conditions frequently describe themselves, in terms that echo neoliberalism, as a "liability."[36]

People who are unemployed are more likely to harm themselves or commit suicide. In one study, they isolated the effects of unemployment as being the cause of suicide (apart from any other predetermining factors) "for one in every 4,200 males who lost their jobs and one in every 7,100 females who lost their jobs."[37] Even before the Great Recession, a midwestern medical examiner's office cited unemployment as the chief cause for suicide in nearly half the files for one year, citing "a 61-year-old man who killed himself after losing his job at a lawn service."[38] Isolated and lonely, workers in the United States experience few supports after unemployment and often seek to take their own lives or do harm to themselves. In other words, workers have limited protection from immediately losing their jobs, whether due to global or local factors, and those who have already lost their jobs, experience significant personal and social distress.

Debt

Real wages for the working class stopped growing in 1973 and have shrunk ever since.[39] At the very same time, mortgage and consumption debt rose in the twenty-first century.[40] When wages stagnated in the 1970s, household debts, including mortgages, were 40 percent of the GDP; by 2005 they reached over 90 percent.[41] Rising housing costs and health care debts, along with booming college tuition costs, were crucial factors in this rise of debtedness. Only a small part of this problem can be laid at the feet of "consumerism" as it is traditionally considered: people living beyond their means. In the late twentieth and early twenty-first century many persons across the globe have fallen into debt in the process of meeting their basic needs.[42]

"Problem debt" has been described as "a condition where a household falls behind in its loan payments and cannot escape the legal consequences of its unmet financial obligations."[43] Although debt often leads to foreclosure, I save the research on foreclosure to the next section.

In a study interviewing persons in Miami-Dade County, social scientists found that "debtor status... was more consistently associated with mental health than any other single traditional indicator of socioeconomic status."[44] In other words, in addition to the research presented here about the links between income and mental distress, debt can be measured separately from socioeconomic status as *its own* stressor. Debt might be one way that the link between socioeconomic status and mental distress is mediated. For example, researchers found that the debt to asset ratio was among the most robust predictors of mental distress.[45] Those in debt reported higher days of mental impairment in the past month than those who were not.[46]

Debt seems to be one link in a chain of adversity, with persons in severe debt less likely to have enough food or medicine.[47] For men, being in debt caused psychological effects beyond simply the perceived consequences of bankruptcy. When controlling for previous mental health problems, researchers found that debt still made a unique contribution to emotional distress.[48]

In terms of consumer debt, older persons facing retirement who had little savings and high debts were much more likely to be depressed. Likewise, those with high consumer debt reported worse physical health, indicating that debt has holistic effects. Those who got high-interest short-term loans were the most likely to become depressed and anxious.[49]

Debt seems to have life- or death-affects. In research at a psychiatric hospital it was found that one third of suicidal patients were in severe debt and those in greater debt had higher suicidal intent. Persons with debt were more likely to be given a psychiatric diagnosis.[50]

Under neoliberalism, large corporations bundle the risky debt of working-class persons and sell it, thus monetizing the suffering of the working class and capitalizing on it. This is one part of what Melinda Cooper calls "debt imperialism," or the aggressive pursuance of the debt of others as part of financial practices.[51] To date, little has been done to prosecute the fraud of those who invested heavily in the insecure debt of others during the financial crisis.[52] As we have seen in this section, problem debt contributes to a distinctive form of psychic suffering, and that such distress can have life-or-death consequences. Already marginalized persons are likely to be saddled with this debt. Another consequence of this research is that investors can benefit from investing in the debt of others, thus owning a share of widespread suffering.

Foreclosure

Predatory lending and speculative investment lead to a well-known housing bubble in the early twenty-first century where many people were living in homes they could not afford. The adjustable rate mortgages (ARM) marketed aggressively to working class and predominantly minority families in the mortgage bubble[53] contributed to a specific kind of psychic distress. Researchers found that those with "high interest debt repayment structures" were more likely to fall physically ill and suffer mental distress.[54] Borrowing money against their mortgages in lines of credit and "cash-out refinancing" became common practices, which accounted for the concerning debt-to-savings ratio.[55]

This lead to a crisis in housing foreclosure, which spiked in 2009 and 2010 with more than 2.8 million homes in foreclosure.[56] Although the housing situation has improved, the impact of foreclosure on working-class families can be long term, leading to later financial difficulties.[57] The mental suffering from foreclosure was felt differently for men and women, since for women, the most severe psychic consequences seem to relate to the stress of multiple moves coming from foreclosure.[58]

A researcher who has focused on the psychic impact of foreclosure has argued that housing foreclosures have had the most profound impact on the mental health of African American communities in the United States. How did this work? The stress from debt was highest for families with many dependents who lived in an area where housing was depreciating. It was lowest for those whose homes were appreciating and who had disposable income. Homes depreciated faster in African American communities and disposable income was also lower, leading to deep widespread distress. He concluded that the impact of housing foreclosure was broadly felt, since it was a "community level stressor...associated with the mental health of all residents," homeowners, and renters combined.[59] The foreclosure crisis added a half-a-day per month of "mentally unhealthy days" between 2006 and 2011.[60] It is unclear the social mechanisms through which this distress was communicated, but the housing crisis clearly added disproportionate stress to communities that had already been harmed by predatory lending practices. Thus, there is a collective dimension to the experience of debt, as the prevailing rate of indebtedness, measured against the stability of the housing market in a given geographical area, impacted psychological distress.[61]

Unemployment, debt, and foreclosure formed a chain of adversity during the Great Recession from which many individuals and families have never recovered. These stressors compounded one another, making it difficult for persons to get much needed help in other areas.[62] Such stresses lead to measurable psychic suffering, including suicide. It is important to note that these forms of psychic suffering were incurred while people were simply trying to survive, making ends meet, putting children through college, and taking care of the elderly, hence much of this mental suffering resulted from economic stress rather than preceding it.[63] In other words, we can see that there is significant psychic stress that comes from the economic conditions of our times, rather than stemming from preexisting mental problems. In the next section we explore *how* economic suffering leads to emotional distress.

Stress, Trauma, and Causation

Carl Walker in the United Kingdom has proposed a stress pileup argument for how economic factors impact mental suffering. In his theory, depression occurs because of exposure to potentially stressful events combined with a reduction of the sources of support to deal with these stresses. He argues that poorer persons are exposed to frequent disruptions, like "bereavement, moving house, social alienation, employment difficulties, the breakdown of a relationship."[64] Described elsewhere as the pileup of "role stress"[65] and painful life events, researchers found that female sole parents in a poor neighborhood in the United Kingdom were more likely to face "humiliating and entrapping" life events that then lead to depression.[66] Using this data Walker maintains that childhood and adulthood stress is one of the key pathways that translate material inequity into mental illness. According to this theory, persons who in lower socioeconomic status positions more frequently face the pileup of stress in their lives, lack resources that wealthier persons might have to cope with such stress, and thus suffer more debilitating results from such exposure.

I maintain that it is important to add the environmental conditions of living in poverty to the stress theory in order to create a more complex picture. There are "socially determined physical and chemical risk and protective factors linked to poverty and inequality such as poor housing, poor diet, drugs, environmental and workplace hazards, injuries, poor transportation, lack of access to quality health care, or physical violence" and these also may contribute to mental distress.[67] Recent research has underscored how persons from a low socioeconomic position are disproportionately affected by environmental harm, which is concentrated in low-income "sacrifice zones."[68]

Researchers emphasized that objective poverty, measured by socioeconomic status was a more robust correlation with mental illness than subjective self-reports of relative poverty. While we are not certain of the exact mechanisms by which financial suffering leads to emotional distress, it is clear that it contributes directly to suffering.

Some researchers have questioned whether poverty causes mental illness (causation) or whether people who are mentally ill drift into more extreme poverty (drift). Evidence is weighted toward the fact that poverty causes mental distress, including studies that control for previous mental illness,[69] although both factors seem to be important.[70] I maintain that however we might settle the causation/drift debate, we must be oriented toward preventing such suffering whenever possible.

28 • Pastoral Power Beyond Psychology's Marginalization

In the United Kingdom researchers examined how mental health was impacted by factors such as owning a home or car, being able to pay bills and being free from financial strain, and found that "poor material standard of living" accounted for "nearly one quarter of all cases."[71] These material approaches indicate that even if it is difficult to capture precisely how economic suffering leads to mental distress, it is possible to isolate precisely how much does so. Since economic conditions are not fixed, but liable to be changed by social policy, I call this percentage *the extent of avoidable suffering brought about by economic causes*. Our share of this suffering as a society has increased in the last several decades. In the next section I explain why.

Four Decades of Inequity: A Neoliberal Project

Social class is a name for how, in US society, different groups have access to limited and valued goods and how they remain at fairly stable levels in terms of their access to these goods. In the last several decades

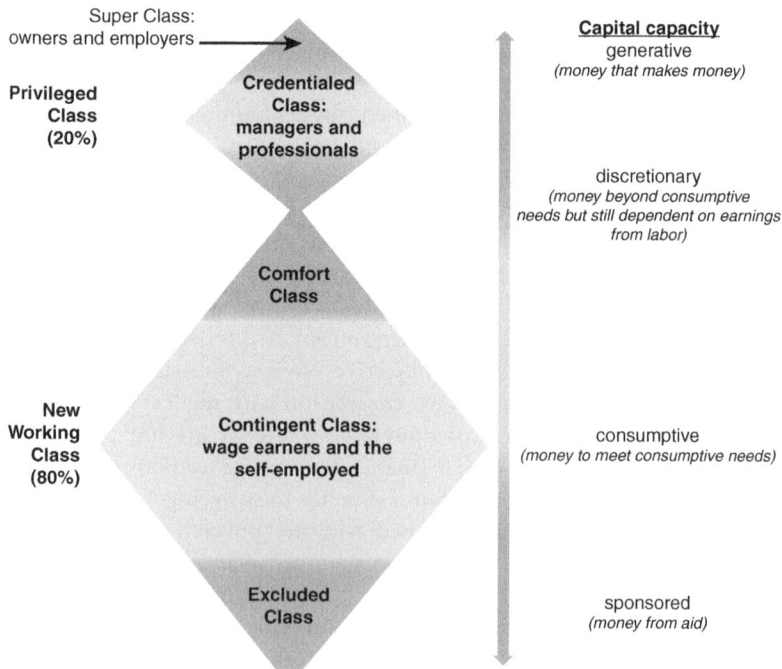

Figure 1.1 The Disappearance of the Middle Class[72]

the financial distance between these groups has grown exponentially as part of a social project called neoliberalism.

One way of exploring this is by looking at income. The real (inflation-adjusted) incomes of working-class Americans—the "nonsupervisory" workers who make up three-quarters of the US workforce—peaked in 1973. The size of the upper class (with incomes over $25 an hour) and lower class (with incomes under $8 an hour) each grew five percentage points in the years from 1973 to 1999, while the size of the middle class (with incomes between $8 and $25 an hour) shrunk by six percent. While many people believe in the notion of a robust working class, what we actually have in the United States is a large working class, as depicted by the double diamond in figure 1.1.

In 1992, a production worker brought home "$1,581 *less* in real income" than in 1973.[73] This trend continued and by 2000 the top ten percent got nearly a third of the national income, the top 20 percent nearly half, while the poorest 20 percent had only five percent of the national income and the poorest ten percent a mere two percent.[74] These shifts in income were accompanied by shrinking benefits, pensions, and employee health care. Additionally, there are more contingent workers than ever and half as many workers are unionized.[75]

Wealth is more important than income since it tells a more complex story about social class. The top five percent has 68 percent of the nation's wealth and the top 20 percent keeps 91 percent of the nation's wealth, leading to a situation where money is kept by a few rather than circulating through the economy.[76] The shift in wealth has also had a gender and racial slant, so that in 2007, before the Great Recession, single Hispanic women had household wealth—excluding vehicles—of $120, and single black women had household wealth of $100.[77] The most persistently poor counties in the United States are in rural rather than urban areas.[78]

These broad differences in income and wealth have been the result of social-class redistribution. These changes were not incidental, but they have taken place as the result of specific policies meant to roll back the Great Society programs of the 1960s and 1970s.[79] In the postwar period there was greater access to valued resources for the middle class in the United States, but in the 1970s elites began to be nervous about their shrinking percentage of the American wealth and instituted policies to redistribute wealth back to the owner class. They controlled the conversation about this by keeping media and education outlets in elite hands.[80] It is unfair to accuse activists of engaging in class warfare when they discuss income inequity since class warfare has already been occurring for some time.[81]

In order for this to work, there had to be a shift in discourse that constructed extreme wealth as natural for some and blamed the poor for using the social safety net. The name for this new discourse was *neoliberalism*. Neoliberalism is a theory that proposes human flourishing is best fostered by liberating markets to function with few restrictions.[82] On the one hand, neoliberal ideology operates as a political force, and on the other hand it serves as a shorthand philosophy. This economic philosophy was instituted by Reagan and others who developed the notion of a liberated and beneficial free market. This philosophy relied on the premise that if money was redistributed to the elites, it would trickle-down to the rest of the population, leading to net benefits for all.[83] Under neoliberalism the market is the dominant institution.

Globalization has been one face of neoliberalism, with tremendous wealth increases for corporations who are moving their industries abroad, quick flows of capital around the world, and aggressive policies by the International Monetary Fund and the World Bank to pressure poor countries through indebtedness to submit to neoliberal policies such as deregulation. Along with the eroding of union powers, this has meant that poorly paid service sector jobs are often the only jobs left in the United States. As Carl Walker summarizes, "globalization has come to represent the decline of unionization, low wages, flexibility, corporate deregulation, welfare bias, increased poverty and an upwardly distributive bias in national economic policy."[84] Yet globalization has often been confused as the cause for neoliberalism. Instead, it followed from the governmental philosophy and its principles: if a philosophy of shared collective responsibility had been in place rather than neoliberalism, some of the excesses of globalization may have been curbed.

Neoliberalism is a philosophy of personal responsibility and initiative. Everyone should be able to pull themselves up by their bootstraps. It presumes equal footing and shared opportunity. The feeling of a neoliberal era is the constant pressure to succeed, a high degree of technological advancement, but fewer resources for the common good and an erosion of the social safety net. In a time of personal responsibility, counseling theories also tend to emphasize solutions within help and people become responsible for themselves.[85] Yet as we saw in the first part of the chapter, the emotional tenor of these times is of increasing suffering. Given the links between poverty and mental illness, it would make sense if these changes of neoliberalism have lead to unnecessary mental suffering.

Neoliberalism was invented to justify redistributing wealth to the elite classes. The invention required blaming the poor for their problems and radically dismantling the social safety net, including programs that addressed mental illness. It is necessary to deconstruct and reverse neoliberalism to address the widespread emotional distress of our times.

Erik Olin Wright's Class Analysis

An important tool for the deconstruction of neoliberalism is a Neo-Marxist class analysis. Erik Olin Wright's Neo-Marxist class analysis does not presume that all societies should become socialist, but rather insists that more egalitarian relationships are possible. He has explained how social class refers to a set of relationships between workers, professionals, and business owners. As Wright summarizes, "Even if 'classlessness' is unachievable, 'less classness' can be a central political objective, and this still requires challenging capitalism."[86]

There are three important conditions of social class in a capitalist economy that can help us understand social justice and worker rights as well as the psychological and social consequences of being in the working class. First, the profits of business owners depend on depriving workers. Second, workers are excluded from some important resources. Third, this exclusion allows owners to take the effort of the working class and use it to their advantage, which is "transfer of the fruits of labor from one group to another."[87] For economic *exploitation* to occur the last category is necessary.

Any discussion that describes classes as occupying different strata on a social ladder based on income or education misses an important point: workers and owners are linked through the process of exploitation in which the fruits of workers' labor are taken from them. This is significant because it gives workers the power to organize and advocate for more equitable work conditions and remuneration.

Social class is not a noun but an adjective, suggesting that people are working class-in-relationship with the owning class. What makes Wright's account so compelling is that he shows the grounds for challenging the unjust appropriation of income to the elite class under neoliberalism. In other words, we are not talking about charity for the poor, but rather a greater share of the fruits of one's own labor, which has been exploited. He also notes that consent must be produced among the working class so they work harder for less gain. Neoliberal ideology that depicts wealth as a natural right or the working poor as "double dippers, cheats, and shirkers" is part of the discourse that produces consent by splitting the middle class between deserving and underserving poor, stigmatizing the use of the social safety net.[88] Workers and owners need each other and this interdependence creates conditions for creating more just working conditions: neoliberal discourse attempts to deny this connection.

Of course, a simple worker–owner dichotomy is not complex enough to account for persons who find themselves in the middle, but who, in this schema, are still linked to the dynamics of production and exploitation. Managers exert authority over workers and get paid an *authority* rent for the emotional toll that it takes on them to do so. Professionals get paid a *skills* rent for the valued credentials or expertise they hold. In each case, they have a *contradictory class location,* that is, they share elements of both owning class and working-class experience.[89]

If we followed a strictly income-based approach to class, we might think that the more money one had, the less likely one would be to suffer from mental distress. A study of more than three thousand participants in the Baltimore area who were interviewed in the 1980s and 1990s showed new findings on social class. Specifically, research led by Carles Muntaner and his colleagues showed that Wright's Neo-Marxist class framework explains that it was actually one's class position, rather than simple income, that correlated with a rise in mental distress.

In order to measure Wright's Neo-Marxist approach to class, Muntaner and his colleagues added three questions about social class pertaining to a diagnostic interview. These questions distinguished "*managers* who have power over subordinates and can influence company policy; *supervisors* who have power over subordinates but who do not have influence in policy making, and *workers* who have neither authority nor influence in policy making," and they measured common forms of distress such as depression, anxiety, alcohol, and substance use—measured through tissue tolerance and withdrawal questions—over a 12-month period in these three groups.[90] If more income resulted in better mental health, supervisors should be healthier than workers. The researchers found that low-level supervisors were twice as likely to be depressed than workers and managers, and that they were twice as likely to abuse alcohol as workers. How do we explain these surprising findings?

The researchers demonstrated the mental health effects of being a *contradictory class position.* In these studies, low-level supervisors have worse mental health than their highly skilled workers, but not their less skilled workers, lending credence to the notion that the contradiction of being in different social-class positions in regard to production and labor may have led to the differentials in mental health. In contrast to the *material* measures of distress presented early in the chapter, this is an example of *psychosocial* research that explores the factors relating to work, autonomy, control, and mental health.[91] This study is important because it indicates that there is suffering that is not measurable simply by income, but by the nature of one's work.

Another study in Spain, measuring the social class and mental health of more than three thousand residents, distinguished managers from nonmanagerial supervisors and workers and found that mental health outcomes were worse for low-level supervisors.[92] Once again, this study showed evidence that seemed to point to social-class results rather than simply socioeconomic status. The research found that 15 percent of low-level male supervisors said they had poor mental health in contrast to nine percent of workers and three percent of managers; the researchers argued that the same hypothesis could not be proven for women, partly because of paucity in the data.[93]

Social class explains where you start in economic terms and also what you have to do to keep going. Wright states this in two propositions that explain the continued impact of social class. First, "What you *have* determines what you get." This means that people who already have more access to the sources of production in a given society are likely to continue to get more resources. Second, "What you *have* determines what you *have to do to get what you get*."[94] This means that the conditions of people's work is systematically impacted by their social-class position, namely, to what extent they have ownership over production and the rights and powers that come from this. Maybe we could imagine a world where social class did not matter very much. For example, if everyone got a basic income then these propositions would not apply. Likewise, if there was a continual lottery of wealth and no inheritance, it might make sense to say that we lived in a classless society.

Yet we live in a very different society where social class is omnipresent, even in our discussions of other intersectional identities such as race, gender, sexual orientation, and disability. Class exists in relationship with these other forms of identity but is not reducible to them, and it is necessary to explore them both. In understanding class, I argue that it is important to deconstruct class rather than foster its continuation. While the Black Consciousness Movement raised awareness by claiming, "Black is beautiful" in the 1960s,[95] it makes little sense to say "poor is beautiful" today.

There are several quite practical implications of this kind of analysis. People have an "interest" based in where they are in the relations of labor and production. It might be in the interest of someone in management to avoid a conversation about increasing break time for workers on the floor of a major retailer. Likewise, workers have an interest in improving the conditions under which the fruits of their labor are taken from them. While neoliberal ideology divided people from each other by positioning each individual as an entrepreneur, persons in working-class positions frequently only succeed if they find ways of collaborating. Working- class persons have a shared interest in protecting their bodies and minds, especially because they are often all that they have to continue to labor in the market.

Second, there is something *antagonistic* about a capitalist economy that is inherent to the economic system itself. This means that conflict between classes is not something to be avoided but something to be fostered. Accusations of class struggle are often veiled attempts to keep workers silent.

I argue that people in the professional classes have a unique responsibility as those who are compensated to create knowledge to critique social-class arrangements in favor of greater equity. Counselors belong to the professional class because they have marketable skills and ministers have a religious authority that gives them the power of discourse—an ability to name and describe the kind of suffering that people are facing in the language of faith. Pastoral theologians, for example, frequently craft theories about the inner life and subjective experience, often in relationship with dynamics having to do with gender, race, religion, and culture. Pastoral theologians have the responsibility to include class, a central analytic for interpreting and changing social suffering, and the time is right for doing so.

Once we understand this Neo-Marxist explanation for the rights and powers of social classes, we can advocate for working-class needs even from a contradictory class position. Understanding the interrelationship of social classes means that there is more ground for shared meaning making, solidarity, and advocacy across the classes. The interdependent nature of social classes offers a way of conceptualizing solidarity that could challenge the capitalist system: indeed capitalism can only be challenged by shared power. Pastoral caregivers need to move toward, rather than away from, class conflict.

Likewise, it offers ways of thinking theologically and pastorally about the meaning of work that persons are engaged in and the distinctive forms of suffering that result from that work. For instance, pastoral caregivers can better understand how being a low-level supervisor can contribute to mental illness despite higher wages, suggesting that there was something damaging and painful about having to appropriate the labor of workers yet not having the benefits of decision-making power. Asking questions about the conditions of work and the social suffering that results from being working class, pastoral care can analyze the felt-experience of capitalist exploitation in order to transform it. To conclude, following from Wright's analysis of social class we can define it more completely now as the *interdependent antagonism of production that links classes together by exploiting the surplus of workers primarily to further capitalist profit*.

Desire, Interest, and the Excluded

One of the critiques of the Marxist framework is that it idealizes the qualified and able-bodied worker while denigrating those in the contingent class or who seem perpetually excluded from the economy.[96] These have been variously titled the "excluded class" who do not possess "productively saleable" labor power.[97] Cambridge economist Joan Robinson is reputed to have said: "The one thing worse than being exploited in capitalism is not being exploited."[98] In a recent study, as many as 43 percent of all adults were not in paid work in the United Kingdom, and 15 percent of those described themselves as "disabled."[99] In the United States one in five persons has a disability and more than half of them describe it as severe.[100]

The Marxist framework mentioned previously, which relies upon class mediated by labor and production, may initially seem to leave out this important group who cannot sell their labor in the marketplace. While it is true that Marx offers laborers more of an opportunity to resist and challenge the power used against them, he also privileges skilled and aristocratic laborers over the many, the peasant horde, those who seem permanently excluded from work. To be fair, in his idealistic descriptions of historical materialism, Marx hoped that society would progress to such a point that labor would no longer be the stifling conditions of workers simply fighting to get by, which he described thusly, "from each according to his ability, to each according to his needs."[101]

Persons permanently excluded from the economy feel isolated. Zygmunt Bauman describes how the original "*dangerous classes*" in the asylum or the prison were meant to be rehabilitated, but now a new reality has taken shape. Now the dangerous classes are excluded "*permanently*...being out of a job increasingly feels like a state of 'redundancy'—being rejected, branded as superfluous, useless, unemployable, and doomed to remain 'economically *in*active.'"[102] Many people who are disabled are also poor around the world and have described how they feel like "surplus populations" and "superfluous people."[103] While Marx called them "outcasts" and said that they must be set apart as a reserve force of labor for times of economic expansion, in our times they seem "declassed."[104] Since they are not "exploited" according to the definition offered earlier, they are excluded. Their exclusion defines their position on the periphery or outside of the labor force.

As we can see, becoming disabled can relate to poverty and we have to use intersectional tools to see the oppression in both circumstances at once.[105] In Kimberlé Crenshaw's critique of how racism and sexism rarely overlapped in legal discourse, she noted how the language of women's domination by patriarchy was rarely available to African American women in the legal sphere since it was overshadowed by race. In that article she argued that while racism and sexism "intersect" within African American women's experience, they exist in cultural systems that are prone to respond to only one of these identities at a time.[106] Persons who are excluded from the US economy as workers and producers frequently experience multiple oppressions that each deserves attention. Muntaner and his colleagues, for example, found that "research on the triad of class, gender, and race tends to finds worse psychiatric disorders among members of the groups exposed to the three forms of inequality."[107] Focusing on only one form of identity at a time lacks the conceptual rigor to adequately respond to the complexities of people's lives and situations.

At the level of intersectionality, it is important that socioeconomic factors are included in the analysis of mental illness. Among the most helpful frameworks to analyze these socioeconomic factors is a Neo-Marxist one, yet Neo-Marxism paradoxically excludes from analysis the very groups marginalized by the economic suffering it hopes to explain. Modifying a disability-rights perspective while including the impact of socioeconomic oppression means insisting that a substantial portion of those suffering from mental illness today is suffering needlessly. Bringing these two perspectives together means modifying Marxism based on a thoroughgoing encounter with those who, for the most part, have been excluded from its framework. The irony here is that the conditions of a neoliberal economy are part of what has made them sick, contributing directly to their emotional distress.[108]

Social class refers to the interdependent antagonism of production that links classes together by exploiting the surplus of workers primarily to further capitalist profit. We must expand this framework to describe how social class also *excludes those deemed as nonproducers, multiplying stereotypes about them that come from being outside the capitalist/worker relation*. In capitalist cultures the workers and the unemployed provide counterpoints that are juxtaposed. This does not mean that we need to reject class activism because it does not adequately include those who feel redundant in the new economy. Rather, our framework needs to be expanded to show exactly how these excluded groups function.

I maintain that the gains that are won by social-class struggles, more than the trickle-down economics of the neoliberal era, are likely to positively impact even those who have been excluded from labor relationships. This could lead to gains in income and redistribution and also the redefinition of work away from an exclusively capitalist model of production to a broader conceptual framework of what is worthy and deserving of compensation.

New solidarity can be fostered between disabled workers and those who can sell their labor in the marketplace. Together, these gains can help workers to win what they need to survive and also support family members who may not be employed. Neoliberalism has no imagination for disability because it considers only profitability and efficiency, so it has difficulty imagining these kinds of coalitions. By challenging capitalism we can revise a society that positions some as redundant, arguing that they are not redundant at all, but it is our limited frameworks that have excluded them.

Characteristics and Traits of the Poor

In the previous section I argued that Neo-Marxist class analysis needs to be expanded in order to include the perspective of persons with disabilities and also suggested that class-based activism could still be helpful for excluded groups. In this section, I explain the meanings of the excluded class in popular imagination by focusing on how neoliberalism has used the discourse of the poor *as an identity* to further legitimate the extreme wealth of the rich. As I have argued previously, the excluded class becomes the negative image against which the worker is pitted and thus a screen upon which the worker's own disempowerment is projected. Constantly reminded that using the social safety net is a sign of weakness, workers are incited to believe in individual merit and the ability to climb the ladder toward success, even while this climb is increasingly impossible for many.

A deeply held notion in the United States is that if an individual fails to succeed, it must be due to a fault that is rooted in some trait within his personality or character. On the other side of the fault equation is the merit one: in a meritocracy everyone is supposed to be able to climb the ladder and amass material wealth. If anything, working-class people typically hold this position more strongly than the elite class.[109]

Sociologist Heather E. Bullock has shown how attitudes about the poor are rooted in the so-called American dream, "the promise that all Americans have a reasonable chance to achieve success as they define it... through their own efforts, and to attain virtue and fulfillment through success."[110] Yet, "Children from low-income families have only a one percent chance of reaching the top five percent of income... children of rich have about a twenty-two percent chance."[111] The gap between the wealthy and the poor is maintained by continually propping up the myth of the American dream.

If the American dream is available to all, but so few achieve it, then one possible way of explaining this is that there is some fault or flaw of the poor that makes it impossible for them to achieve middle-class standards. Children are socialized to prefer trait-based descriptions of poverty.[112] In one study, 8 to 17-year-olds were asked to describe the poor. Eight-year-olds tended to use concrete descriptions that referred to appearance and possessions while 17-year- olds described abilities and traits that pertained to the poor's character. White middle-class teens in a Denver suburb who were shown pictures of persons that were described as poor, neutral, or rich, offered different characteristics of each. "Although poor strangers were rated as working harder and as more generous, they were also judged to steal more often, feel worse about themselves, and make friends less easily than neutral or wealthy strangers."[113] Likewise, "Wealthy strangers were perceived as being more intelligent, more likely to be successful, and happier than poor or neutral strangers."[114] Young people are socialized into trait-based descriptions of poor people and these descriptions help provide a justification for poverty.

Matthew Hunt made a series of significant explorations into beliefs about wealth and poverty that indicated that African Americans and Latinos were less likely to make individualistic attributions for poverty than whites, but they were still very likely to make individualistic attributions for wealth—"a remarkable consensus appears to exist on the issue of individualistic beliefs about wealth"—and this is surprising given how wealth is often transmitted intergenerationally through investments and property.[115] The belief in the meritocracy has surprisingly enduring effects, despite evidence that disproves it.

Since many in the United States believe in the American Dream and the myth of meritocracy, this makes it difficult to talk directly about how social class works. Even young children are taught to see the poor as having definable traits that help explain their poverty. Likewise, among marginalized groups there is a sense that the rich must have earned their wealth. By deconstructing the myth of the equal playing field, it is possible to argue for more just arrangements for persons in the working and excluded class, critiquing the unjust compensation of the top one, five, and ten percent, as well as the ways these groups hold onto inherited wealth. Likewise, by addressing and deconstructing these myths of natural rights to wealth, we deconstruct the stigma and shame surrounding poverty and also have new lenses with which to appropriate the social science research on social class.

Media outlets and politicians constantly repeat tropes about the traits and attributes of the working and excluded classes. Poor people are frequently described as having a discernable and definable culture that separates them from everyone else. When anthropologist Oscar Lewis first described a "culture of poverty" in which people would not stand up and resist their oppression, he could likely not have perceived how Democrats and Republicans would use this trope decades later alike to defund the social safety net program of income subsidies.[116]

Bullock also includes an intersectional component of her analysis. Although poverty cuts across all sectors of society, she argues that media-overrepresentation of the poor as black and female creates hypervisibility of poverty among African Americans and invisibility of poverty among whites, supporting stereotypes in the minds of whites. This makes it easier for the dominant racist culture to link together poverty and race, justifying negligent approaches to each.[117]

One way to keep up the myth of a discernable culture for the poor is to study the families of the poor and their relationships for signs of dysfunction. In her definitive treatment of the subject, Alice O'Connor maintains that the characteristics of poor families are being mistaken as the causes of poverty. At the same time, structural explanations of economic inequity have disappeared from poverty research.[118] O'Connor linked this trend with an individualizing tendency in modern social science research that goes back to a several-centuries old goal, that of discerning the deserving from the undeserving poor.[119] This can be seen in the poverty research funded through government organizations such as the Office of Economic Opportunity and associated think tanks. The notion that the poor have definable traits that make them responsible for their plight is reinforced by social science research that, since Reagan's presidency, has exhaustively studied the characteristics and attributes of the poor.

The transformation from social structural explanations for poverty to personal-individual explanations can sometimes be symbolized by a single term. In his book *The War against the Poor,* Herbert Gans showed how the term "underclass" came to do such heavy explanatory work. The term was coined by Gunner Myrdal and originally referred to those excluded from society, much as my term "excluded class" has served in the foregoing section.[120] Nevertheless, with its appropriation by Charles Livermore as a racial and behavioral term, it began to be used to describe the violence and the terrorizing behavior of gangs. The term became popularized in major magazines in the 1970s and 1980s and was linked with language such as "intergenerational, biological (or genetic), and hereditary," and even "hardcore."[121] Gans argues that the underclass was seen as black, since "poor whites have almost never been described as underclass in the national media."[122] The term underclass appeared an average of 90 times a year in the *New York Times* between 1985 and 1993, peaking in 1989. This occurred at the beginning of the neoliberal era. While the term refers to economics 44 percent of the time in the 1970s by the 1990s the term referred to behavior 44 percent of the time, with only four percent of its instances referring to economics.[123] According to Gans, the war against the poor is waged as a war of words, and the term underclass has brought together multiple discourses of race, gender, criminality, deviance, and delinquency. By playing on racial and gender oppression the media implicitly blames and stigmatizes the poor, according to Gans.

Understanding the discourse used against the poor is a significant part of changing attitudes toward the concept of social class and crafting more substantial solidarity for the working and contingent classes. Neoliberalism has employed discourse such as the underclass to depict the poor as a particular kind of people. Just as a philosophy of personal responsibility came to dominate the public discourse in the United States, poor people began to be studied to discover their discernable culture and what it was in their family structure that made it more likely for them to be poor. As a result, people are likely to mistake the *traits* and *qualities* of family life in working-class communities as a cause for their poverty. Rather, it is the symptom of living without access to adequate resources, including food, shelter, transportation, education, and other important goods.

Discourse about working-class persons plays on an implicit racism—you should care about poverty because white people are poor as well—and at the same time this research does not seem to address the entrenched nature of economic factors, as described previously in the section on social class. Gans, for example advocates "debunking" classism by challenging prejudicial attitudes toward the poor.[124] Bullock insists that simply understanding these statistics can lead to change among those with good intentions who can help deconstruct stereotypes about the poor. Yet it is clear that simply a fresh language about the poor will not suffice, as if to say that new terminology would make widespread and long-term suffering disappear.

Paradoxically, if the new economy is more likely to make people suffer mental distress, it is also more likely to make them feel responsible personally for their mental illness. Just as a neoliberal philosophy pervaded government, mental health care became deinstitutionalized so those who had been impacted by economic stress were left homeless, institutionalized in prisons, or required to fend for themselves. People who become mentally ill, in part because of the stress from the new economy, are at an intersectional disadvantage—they become less likely to get work and further marginalized.

The goal of much poverty discourse is to make working-class persons into "others" for the professional and elite classes so that they will be unable to see our common cause with them and develop our shared interest. Once positioned as a discernable culture, the working-class are seen through the lens of pathology. When mental distress enters the picture, the stigma against mental illness combines with the stigma against poverty to create a double injury to identity. What needs to be recovered, then, is the understanding of how the concerns of the working class impact all of us in US society, and how we are directly affected by what happens to the working class even as we participate in our economic system.

A Critically Engaged Collective Responsibility

The purpose of the research presented here is to foster social transformation rather than simply to raise awareness about more respectful socially aware pastoral counseling. In this way we seek the tools to critique the unnecessary suffering of a capitalist system and offer a more humane social system. In this approach we offer the model of solidarity for pastoral care and counseling. Discovering a shared interest across class positions means working to change the conditions of work, what one has to do to survive, and also foregrounding the *voice* of those who are in working-class positions. It is impossible to have true solidarity without equal participation.

Even in proposing this we must be aware that there are some who struggle to be working class and who find that they cannot offer marketable labor. Since they cannot gain entrance to shared working-class interest, it can be difficult to develop anything like a "class consciousness" for those within an excluded-class position, unless one depends upon a broader ethical, religious, and humanistic basis for shared advocacy. Yet such cross-class friendships must often occur in order for the excluded class to have their voices heard; this is different from a model of charity in which an undeserved gift is bestowed as a grace from a more able person toward another; it is rather a reflection of the demands of justice based on an intuition of common humanity that challenges the reduction of a person to the object of someone's care or a means to an end.

This deep solidarity can be perhaps most difficult in relationship with those who have already faced the stigma of mental illness that stems from the very socioeconomic stressors that burdened them. All too often social scientists are cynical about the outcomes from their research and the data leads to new theories but the same social conditions. The belief held by many in the field of mental health is "that most social outcomes, including mental health, reflect personal autonomous choices [so] . . . there is little that society, as a whole, is obliged to do for persons who are afflicted by mental disorders."[125] Muntaner and his colleagues contrast this personal responsibility model with a more integrated image of social oppression and collective responsibility. In one study, the so-called liberals were able to feel empathy for homeless persons but felt little obligation to change their situation. By contrast, these researchers suggest that a "structural" view that "focuses on social relations of class, race, ethnicity, and gender inequality" can include more "collective responsibility."[126] Incidentally, this feeling of collective responsibility is found more among African American men than among white working-class men.[127]

Muntaner and his colleagues conclude, "There is nowadays sufficient evidence to suggest that class, gender, and racial/ethnic inequalities in mental health stem from social structures, rather than solely from personal choices or individual attributes."[128] If social factors such as economic inequality play a strong role in how mental illness expresses itself, and if these factors can be changed, then it is our communal responsibility to transform them. It will only be possible to change the core conditions of suffering in our time when we have changed the conditions that have produced this suffering and maintained it.

Outlining the research on the impact of being in the working-class position, it is fair to say that being denied access to necessary goods in their life actively harms people in this class position. This harm has a psychic impact and it affects the fabric of social relationships. Without an analysis of this damage, it is impossible to move forward and propose feasible solutions. This is quite different from saying that the harm of poverty comes from the social or psychic makeup of the poor, who through their definable culture have no ability to organize or defend their social position.

It is possible to offer a range of adjustments to the system, for example, suggesting that various models of "uplift" occurs so that the working class joins the ranks of the professional classes, yet most of these adjustments do not deal with the core conditions of capitalism and the harm that it causes. Many solutions to the problem of capitalism offer readjustments to income inequity as the solution.

Theologian Joerg Rieger has argued that this is akin to treating symptoms without addressing the cause. Developing more rigorous alternatives means offering critiques that are more thoroughgoing and address the roots of labor, property, and power as seen in social-class analysis. Likewise, it is impossible to prop up an unsustainable system, since the degradations of neoliberal capitalism have also affected the planet. With Rieger's recent publication of *Religion, Theology, and Class* a model of solidarity is proposed that takes seriously the conditions of labor in a Neo-Marxist framework and also centers the work of transformation on solidarity with the working class, a solidarity that now has a broader basis than ever before.[129]

Rieger maintains that much suffering is indeed *intersectional*, but that social-class analysis can help us build new coalitions. A thorough awareness of class oppression helps us see many of the fraught issues of our times, whether access to the rights to marry or illegal immigration, are also struggles that have to do with people's social class-in-relationship with others. He argues that understanding class has the potential to lead to "deep solidarity"[130] since "black and white workers have more in common with undocumented workers from south of the US border...than with the rich."[131] I would add that, given the size of the new working class in the double-diamond diagram mentioned earlier, many persons share interests with working-class persons even if they had thought of themselves as middle class or professional class. What this means is not subordinating all other identities to class but seeing how the production of identities has often reified forms of difference to the exclusion of discussing the painful realities of poverty and economic oppression.[132]

Erik Olin Wright has argued that social scientists cannot be neutral but must offer solutions to address the problems that they study. He argues that social science research should be geared toward emancipatory aims, and he maintains that social systems frequently cause harm to persons. By understanding these social systems, researchers must work to alleviate the harm, also providing tools to ameliorate this suffering. He names his normative moral presumption that "all persons should have broadly equal access to the necessary material and social means to live flourishing lives" as well as the ability "to participate meaningfully in decisions about things which affect their lives."[133]

Some of his ideas are not new. For example, he offers alternatives to capitalism such as "universal basic income"—the old rubric of negative tax that was no longer studied once neoliberalism took over in the United States—that would be paired with basic health care and education as an equal right.[134] While resisting our tendency to blame capitalism for all our ills, he offers a potential solution as a form of "community…any social unit within which people are concerned about the well-being of other people," a condition that he says is intensely contradicted by capitalism.[135] Wright calls for a reenvisioning of the social good that would think broadly about how rights and necessities could be met in ways that fostered human community and flourishing, encouraging responsiveness to one another's needs. Such reflection has been echoed by Jung Mo Sung in a recent article asking for a "greed line" to be established in upper-level incomes that would limit the accumulation of wealth at the top.[136]

Pastoral Theology Interpreting a Neoliberal Era

This chapter began with the story of Jackie Stanley, who, despite all that she had done to reinvent herself, felt like a failure in the twenty-first century and blamed herself for not working hard enough. The second couple interviewed in *Two American Families,* the Newmans, also struggled following a job layoff. The husband Tony, lost his job and was unable to secure a similarly paying position. He took low-wage jobs and had to work at odd hours. The wife, Terry, began working various jobs to make ends meet, but their different schedules led to conflict in their marriage. The Newmans were a white Catholic family, and they found their faith to be an important resource to them. Their priest even invited the family to the altar when Tony got a new job, showing that the entire community of faith has been supporting them through the struggle of unemployment. Yet throughout the film, through the parent's divorce and the foreclosure of their home, the family becomes less observant.

Claude Stanley, Jackie Stanley's husband, was a minister in his church and he talked about how God was the most important support to him through times of struggle. He preached often about how significant it was to continue to praise God, even during times of trial. God is what helped the Stanleys survive and interpreting God's blessings through Scripture and worship each week helped find support to move through difficult times. As we can see, religion has played a significant role in peoples' lives during the era of neoliberalism and during the economic downturn. Religious leaders and communities of faith are often called upon to directly address the economic suffering in their communities.

Counselors are also called upon for help. As they experienced the stress of much lower wages and an inability to make their mortgage payment, the Newmans went through a difficult time in their family life and saw a marriage therapist. In a scene in the documentary, Terry Newman and her daughter discuss the daughter's reluctance to go to the therapist and her skepticism regarding the therapist's ability to help them. The daughter says, "He's always so serious. It's always about *tell me your problems.*" The mother responds by stating "He's just trying to get down to the problem."[137] What the daughter seems to suggest is that the counselor's categories of problems do not fit the real circumstances of their lives. It's the conditions of work and the stresses of labor that bare down on this family, not generations of pathological dysfunction or mistaken cognitive beliefs.

Ministers and counselors are frequently invited to travel with persons in the story of their lives through experiences of despair and distress. At times, they are even called upon to interpret that suffering. It is clear that clergy are approached first for mental health care in many communities, and so have a role to play in helping persons understand what they are going through.[138]

Michel Foucault described the phenomenon of *pastoral power* as that ability to hold together the one and the many in community, individually attending to the "economy of souls" even as one travelled with the entire flock of the faithful. There are signs that the Stanleys and the Newmans access their faith as an important part of their support system, and they use counselors in the community to help them interpret their suffering. For Foucault there were "border practices" within ministry that can be especially helpful during times of economic oppression—*mysticism,* communicating to persons that they are seen and known by God, *community*—pledging care and solidarity to one another, *asceticism*—sacrificing for one another for the sake of the common good, *Scripture*—confirming through interpretation God's presence, and *eschatology*—giving hope through reminders that the current social arrangements of power are temporary. He indicated that these practices could challenge current power arrangements and were especially helpful to the marginalized in a given society. I return to these themes in chapter 5.

Drawing from Foucault's notion of pastoral power, I maintain that it includes the capacity to interpret a person's suffering with them, when one is invited to do so. Pastoral power is strengthened if a minister shares elements of the same culture and experience, is deepened if the minister is invited to help interpret one's story, and is fostered if the minister can travel with a person for a longer period of time. Thus *pastoral power* consists of three elements—shared experience, an invitation to interpret, and a temporal element.

There are two significant tasks for ministers interpreting the intense suffering of economic oppression in the twenty-first century. First, attending to that suffering means resisting internal attribution of blame or shame for what are, quite often, socially caused factors. Since anxiety or depression may have come about secondary to job loss or the pressures of problem debt and unemployment, that mental suffering is not one person's responsibility. Including this economic component can be challenging, since in the African American community, clergy are often sought for counseling, but people hesitate to share financial struggles.[139] In order to engage this task it is important for the caregiver to understand as much as possible about the conditions of economic life that impact daily existence for persons struggling in the new economy.

The second task is to foster active solidarity with the working-class rights issues that would restore class power to those who are suffering. In other words, it is not enough to measure the emotional impact of economic suffering unless we do so with the aim of alleviating it, and not simply in one instance but through addressing the social conditions that make suffering likely to persist. Joining ministerial efforts with advocacy work means that, even as they engage on the front lines interpreting the suffering of the current economic crisis, ministers and counselors can work with advocacy organizations such as Jobs with Justice to advocate for increased workers rights. This approach builds on recent pastoral theological analyses that have called for an element of advocacy to the counselor's role.[140]

The Social Class of Ministry

Ministerial work and counseling practices also have their own social-class location and it is important to understand that location in order to foster more transformative social-class relationships. Clergy frequently answer calls for assistance from persons in their community and face the difficult task of allocating limited congregational funds to meet emergency needs. To ministers it often seems that all they have are small acts of resistance and interpretation to resist the flood of poverty and oppression.

And there are also the contradictions inherent in ministry itself. Ministers are likely to live at or below the material level of the communities where they work.[141] This is even truer for women clergy, who, in some denominations earn a quarter less than their male counterparts for the same work.[142] Given what we have seen from the studies of material measures in the first part of this chapter, this lack of resources, whether in the form of low income or the lack of net wealth, can put chronic stress on ministers and even leave them at risk for mental illness.

In other words, pastors are affected by the same trends of globalization in which capital has been moved elsewhere, and they are forced to care for circumstances that are largely result of income inequities. According to the Bureau of Labor and Statistics, congregational Protestant pastors make an average of $46,000 in income annually. Catholic diocesan priests on the other hand make around $27,000 annually, regardless of the size of their parish.[143] Nevertheless, income varies widely for Protestant congregational pastors, with small- to mid-size churches barely being able to pay their pastor above the poverty threshold.[144] Persons who serve predominantly minority congregations such as African American and Latino congregations often barely make it above the poverty level because of the way that structural poverty has affected these congregations. While mainline denominations offer health care to their clergy, believer-based traditions and free churches frequently do not.[145]

Additionally, pastors frequently leave seminary in debt, with no conceivable way to recoup these losses. "More than a quarter of students graduating in 2011 with a Master of Divinity degree had more than $40,000 in debt from theological education and five percent were more than $80,000 in the red."[146] In this research we have seen how non-mortgage debt created conditions that led to anxiety for many.[147]

In a recent sociological survey of ministry Jackson Carroll argues that one of the chief problems is that the church equates financial success and high memberships with ministerial success, thus replicating the economic logic of neoliberalism. He maintains that the church now has a two-tiered compensation structure but that "many Protestant clergy will not reach the upper tier during their career."[148] According to his research findings, many pastors find themselves occupying two social-class positions at once because they are increasingly bivocational. Bivocational pastors now constitute 18 percent of mainline Protestant churches, 29 percent of conservative Protestant churches, and 41 percent of clergy in traditionally African American denominations.

The upshot of all of this is that church authorities and seminary leaders often operate with an image of ministry that no longer matches the reality that many clergy face: "the large majority of Protestant clergy will almost inevitably spend their entire ministry in small or medium-sized congregations" while the denominational officials and laity operate from an image of a pastor progressing higher and higher up the pyramid, reflective to financial, if not spiritual success.[149]

Little wonder, then, that clergy fall victim to a variety of psychiatric problems during the course of their work. A missing ingredient in pastoral care conversations about self-care is a discussion of economic disempowerment. One pathway for pastors to become mentally distressed is through the fact of chronic economic stress. Given what we learned about material factors such as housing tenure or owning a car directly impacting depression and anxiety, we can see how the stress pastors are under is not just the result of the pastoral care work that they do but the material conditions in which they live. Another pathway for pastors to become mentally distressed is through their perceived inequity in the larger community since this self-comparison can lead to greater depression. According to Rogers-Vaughn, it was the societies with the highest income inequities that had the highest level of depression.[150] The much-touted economic diversity of congregations can also be a liability if vast income inequities in the community lead to depression for some. The gap between clergy income/wealth could be a contributing factor for *clergy* depression—as we have seen from the research, prestige and education alone cannot protect a clergy person from the psychic effects of poverty.

Frequently pastors have expertise and skills—manifested in the professional degree—which set them apart from a strictly working-class position, yet as we have seen the power of this position depends upon having a market for these skills. Indeed, in a strict social-class sense, the "symbolic power" of these skills would not be enough if they did not lead to some more privileged position in class relations.[151] For this to occur, pastors would have to receive some "skill rent" based on the advanced preparation that they have had, as Wright describes, "a wage above the costs of producing and reproducing their labor power."[152] In order for their position as experts to translate into true class power they would have to control limited knowledge and thereby a scarce form of labor power. Since pastors occupy a complex class position, experts attempting to sell their skills in a market in which their labor is increasingly devalued, they are even more strikingly exposed to the rapid changes in income inequity described earlier. Ministers need a living wage and health care and access to the same goods that the working class require. Since church giving is at Depression-era levels, the social position of pastors is thereby linked explicitly to the economic changes that have occurred under neoliberalism.[153]

Pastors increasingly occupy the lower echelons of what Perrucci and Wysong called the "comfort" working class, skilled workers who were not able to invest. At the same time, clergy are prepared with the skills and credentials that should seem to land them higher in the income stratification. What this means, in Wright's terms, is that clergy occupy a "contradictory class position" but one that is not subsidized by any clear "skills rent" or "authority rent" since their work is increasingly not covering the cost of their education. Understanding this pattern sheds light on the fact that clergy have a great deal to lose during a time of economic downturn.

This may lead to the kind of advocating and organizing for social change that attempts to bring a broad base of material necessities to more persons in the US society, leading to solidarity among the *de facto* working class where clergy are positioned. This could also lead to the kind of imagination that could help clergy identify with the excluded class and advocate for their needs. Unfortunately, it is also possible that pastors would use their power to identify upward as a way to both secure support for the ongoing ministries of the church and also foster their own social position. Rieger has noted the phenomenon that many parish boards are made up of persons exclusively from middle- and upper-class positions.[154]

Conclusion

Ministers hear the stories of the Stanleys and the Newmans of their communities every day. As they do so, they witness the rise in anxiety and distress and other kinds of mental suffering brought about by the current economic situation. Along with the lack of resources there is also, under a neoliberal framework, increasing pressure to lift oneself up by one's bootstraps, so economic suffering can be interpreted as a sense of personal failure.

When a minister begins helping a working-class family to talk about their problems, she might begin to think of that family as "disorganized" and "dysfunctional" unless she considers the complex sources of oppression bearing down upon the family. Listening in such cases requires resisting stereotypes about the culture of poverty.

Through the research presented in this chapter, it is clear that mental distress from the Great Recession and the broader neoliberal era is widespread and this suffering invites ministers to imagine what things are like for the working class. While ministers may be tempted to identify with professional and elite classes in their communities, their own *contradictory class position* means it is necessary for them to join their interest with the working class in their communities. What happens to Jackie Stanley may eventually impact them.

Such a social-class imagination must also attend to the excluded class, those who perceive that they are no longer able to sell their labor in the marketplace. From this perspective, seeing the suffering that has happened to them as a result of economic injustice and crafting conditions in which they can be more fully included is a central task of the church.

Through this chapter we have traced the changes through the last four decades of the social project of neoliberalism. This project has systematically redistributed income and goods to the elite class in our society. Keeping this reality in mind means that we must look for social and structural solutions to problems that have individual effects. Even as we do so, we must actively resist the tendency to blame individuals and communities for their suffering.

Accessing some of the neglected insights from our social science tradition, namely material from social psychiatry that explores the impact of the social world on the mental health of entire societies, means that we can interpret mental distress differently and treat it more effectively.

In the next chapter I discuss how the rise of a medical model of mental illness has coincided with the changes described as neoliberalism in this chapter. This means that just as social conditions of inequity have heightened, the medical model used to describe emotional distress has become ascendant. Descriptive psychiatry, exemplified in third and subsequent editions of the Diagnostic and Statistical Manual, reads mental illness as a list of symptoms that can be seen in the behavior of an individual. A pharmaceutical industry markets compounds that are "good drugs" for people's suffering, while other drugs are penalized. Looking at the biomedical complex, we see how a mental illness diagnosis can pathologize suffering by placing in the brain and genes of individuals what is inherently the result of their social oppression. Challenging this interpretation means resisting individualism in favor of collective options for addressing the oppression that comes from economic suffering.

I maintain that Jackie Stanley and those like her in her community are not failures, but persons worthy of dignity and created in the Image of God. Likewise, the Newman's marriage relationship was not plagued by some kind of deficit or dysfunction but by the daily realities of having to struggle to survive even while raising three children. It is possible for people to discover this for themselves in a ministerial relationship, the kind in which the counselor attends to the social world and its economic ramifications. Fostering a pastoral counseling approach that directly addresses economic suffering means knowing as much as possible about the contextual causes of such suffering.

The condition of working-class suffering is directly linked to the economy, and much emotional and mental distress is unnecessary. Much of the rise of mental illness in the United States is caused by preventable economic distress.

It also means listening in a way that fosters solidarity, not forging alliances with the most powerful but with those who have been impacted by the downturn. Families such as the Stanleys and Newmans are in need of relationships of advocacy that addresses working-class concerns. What is at stake in this advocacy is no less than what it means to be *pastoral*, namely to believe in a God who requires both love and justice from us and from our social relationships (Micah 6:8).

CHAPTER 2

Psychiatric Power and the Limits of Biomedical Diagnosis

In one of the pastoral care classes during my seminary training, we were discussing the possibility that mental illness may not exist, but may simply be the culture's projection of normality on a person, when my professor responded, "Yet, if you see someone with a mental illness, you just know [that they're sick]." This response did not set well with me, but I began to wonder about what kind of world this comment might imply. Did everyone have this power of definition equally? Those who were able to determine mental illness exercise the power of normative judgment.

The assumed power to discern the pathological from the normal—a presumably great power indeed—has repeatedly been shown faulty in both academic studies and popular lore. For example, a team of top UK psychiatrists performed a battery of tests on a group to determine who had mental illness, but scored with only 50 percent accuracy.[1]

In "On Being Sane in Insane Places," an article published in the journal *Science* in 1973, Stanford psychologist David L. Rosenhan and seven other ostensibly "normal" participants voluntarily committed themselves to mental hospitals all over the country claiming to hear voices.[2] None of the staff suspected that these patients were pretending. Seven participants were diagnosed as schizophrenics and one as manic-depressive. Their average hospital stay was 19 days. Only when they accepted their diagnosis and claimed to still be sick but getting better were they discharged as "in remission."[3] The patients previously diagnosed with mental illness staying on the wards saw them taking notes about their lives on the ward and understood that these pseudopatients were journalists and not mentally ill.

Rosenhan maintains that "psychiatric diagnosis...locates the sources of aberration within the individual...and only rarely within the complex of stimuli that surrounds him [sic]."[4] Once the diagnosis is given, otherwise normal aspects of his or her personality are explained through reference to that diagnosis. In the quote from the "schizophrenic" pseudopatient's case file, what could be considered "normal" aspects of a person's life, such as one's changing relationships with one's parents, are rendered pathological:

> This white 39-year-old male...manifests a long history of considerable ambivalence in close relationships, which begins in early childhood. A warm relationship with his mother cools during adolescence. A distant relationship with his father is described as becoming very intense. Affective stability is absent...And while he says that he has several good friends, one senses considerable ambivalence embedded in these relationships also.[5]

Rosenhan suggests that the clinical language in this case file has superseded what would have been a fairly normal account of a person's life. Such a description is striking to the reader because we know that he is a journalist. Because of the diagnostic label, everyday particulars become scientific data. The changes in this man's emotional life are seen as signs of "ambivalence," a prominent theme of schizophrenic diagnosis during the 1960s and 1970s.[6] Now that he has become a patient his relationships seem to have the quality of "intensity" rather than normalcy. Overall, the scientific account offers explanatory categories to make sense of a person's otherwise unclassified experience.

The new status of patient has more than simply linguistic effects. The pseudopatients reported experiencing verbal abuse and even, in one case, physical abuse on the wards. They were rarely spoken to or heard. Once they became patients, professionals often refused to answer their questions, frequently walking away—a behavior that continues to happen to people diagnosed with mental illness today. This suggests the power of a pathological label—at least in the institutional setting—as it negatively impacts a person's ability to have an influence and power. In evaluating his research at the end of his life, one of Rosenhan's chief claims was that he wished to examine the mental hospital anthropologically and not simply craft a critique of diagnosis.[7] His main concern was how patients were treated on the wards. Some have speculated that the public reaction to the Rosenhan study, along with the demedicalization of homosexuality,[8] contributed to the ascendancy of the third edition of the *Diagnostic and Statistical Manual of Mental Disorders* (DSM-III) approach as an attempt to restore psychiatric validity.[9]

Arthur Kleinman, a significant voice in psychiatric anthropology, argues that each diagnosis is an "interpretation" of an illness experience within a particular social world that recasts the social world in medical terms.[10] In other words, a psychiatric diagnosis replaces the patient's familiar world with an unfamiliar one. He draws attention to the problem, expecting to find a diagnosis that could correspond to a person's experience, when there is such a wide variety of cultural norms that impact the interpretation of that experience. Kleinman suggests that any diagnosis could only be "[verified through] observations in given social systems (a village, an urban clinic, a research laboratory)."[11] What this means is that significant aspects of a person's experience are likely to be lost during the process of diagnosis:

> The professionalization of human problems as psychiatric disorders ... causes sufferers (and their communities) to lose a world, the local context that originates their experience through the moral reverberations and reinforcement of popular cultural categories about what life means and what is at stake in living.[12]

Note that Kleinman suggests that "diagnosis" is inherently cultural and that Western psychiatry shears away a person's context. Diagnosis seems to presume an equivalence that is not there. There is supposed to be a conceptual match between outward behavior and inner reality in a diagnosis, but, contrary to Karl Jaspers' influential *General Psychopathology*, it simply does not work that way since there is no way of mapping directly from the body to science.[13]

Discourse as Productive Truth

How should we understand what Rosenhan calls the "stickiness of diagnostic labels" and how do we make sense of the power that these labels have?[14] One of the most helpful lenses to explain what happens in these studies is *discourse*. According to French philosopher/historian Michel Foucault, discourse is what is written and said that counts as truth in texts, rules, official documents, and situated practices, and also refers to the "rules of formation of statements" or how something is counted to be true.[15] There are two parts of discourse in this definition: what is taken to be true and the implicit logic that justifies given statements as true. This logic makes sense in institutional settings where these discourses are put to use. Certain communities have their own discourses, their rules for speaking, and their justification or legitimation of these rules.

Discourse is not merely speech. Analyzing discourse also involves noticing the silences around what could be said and how these silences are productive of a certain kind of "truth": "There is no binary division to be made between what one says and what one does not say."[16] In discussing the history of sexuality, Foucault notes that "we must try to determine the different ways of not saying... things [about sexuality], how those who can and those who cannot speak of them are distributed, which type of discourse is authorized, or which form of discretion is required."[17] Here we see a meaning-making loop: discourse creates persons especially responsible for deploying discourse and managing it. It also creates silences and these blank spaces are productive vacuums where discourse gathers signification.

Foucault describes the academic disciplines of history, science, philosophy, theology, and psychiatry, as "bearers of discourse" and indicates that psychiatry most often tries to normalize people through discourse, what he describes as a general "medicalization of behaviors, conducts... desires, etc."[18] No single person is responsible for discourse; it circulates in systems and has effects that transcend the intentions of individuals. This is a point worth reinforcing. Powerful cultural and social forces make the discourse of a particular time difficult to perceive, and for this reason it can be hard to hold a single individual responsible for reproducing discourse in any given setting.

Rather than expecting that our language could point directly to hidden truths or inner realities that exist within or behind the language, discourse stresses language's capacity for shaping reality. Therefore, it helps explain the effects of power expressed through language. If language is essentially constructive, then it has different effects in different settings. Words, then, are not neutral signifiers that point directly to an objective referent; rather, they are powerful carriers of meaning that not only signify but also construct reality.

Discourse has incredible power to shape what people expect to see. To return for a moment to the Rosenhan study, he included another part of the experiment, in which he told mental health clinics that he would be sending some pseudopatients to feign symptoms at their clinics. Of a sample of 196 patients, 42 were deemed pseudopatients by staff members, and 23 by psychiatrists; 19 were expected to be pseudopatients by a staff member and a psychiatrist together. Rosenhan sent no pseudopatients to the clinic.

This presents a complication to the idea of the "stickiness of diagnostic labels": if labels are universally sticky then why did mental health experts conclude that some of the patients presenting with complaints were actually healthy? Something more complex is happening at the level of diagnostic thinking. Because of Rosenhan's notification, mental health practitioners were primed to see normalcy rather than pathology (perhaps for the first time!) and for this reason they diagnosed pseduopatients when Rosenhan sent them none. This research suggests that the expectation of mental illness or mental health primes people to find mental illness or mental health. *People with more social, cultural, and economic power will be more likely to be perceived as mentally healthy, while people with less power and wealth will be interpreted as disordered in a variety of ways.*

Discourse has a double referent: it refers to authorized speech and also the contexts that authorize it. Foucault's notion of discourse gives a necessary framework for understanding how psychiatric terminology works in particular institutional settings. With Foucault's discourse lens we have a new principle that can be applied: all diagnoses are context-specific and they are produced and deployed in particular institutional settings. Understanding how shifting cultural frames impact the discourse of psychiatry is crucial to grappling with how we all embody various discourses of disorder in our work, applying them to persons different from us with the result of social control.

Blaming the Victim in an Age of Overmedicalization

Exploring the context-specific dimensions of mental illness is especially important at a time when mental health diagnoses and reported mental distress are on the rise. In 1961, nine percent of Americans received Social Security Disability payments for problems related to mental illness. In 2010, that number rose to 19 percent, roughly one in five Americans.[19] There was a 35-fold increase of mental illness diagnoses for children during the same decades, with one in five children being diagnosed with mental illness in the last year.[20] Depression is supposedly 10 to 20 times more prevalent than it was half a century ago, with children of 14 or 15 seeing the first onset.[21] The rate of suicide has increased 28 percent since 1999.[22] At some point in their lives, 46 percent of Americans met the American Psychiatric Association's criteria for at least one mental illness and 9.6 million, about four percent of the population, report having a mental illness that has caused disruption in their life in the last year.[23]

Yet there are also signs that we describe more and more behavior as mental illness, indicating that we have medicalized emotional distress to an unprecedented degree. There are terms we can use to describe this shift in opinion about mental distress. Sociologist Peter Conrad defined medicalization as "a process by which nonmedical problems become defined and treated as medical problems, usually in terms of illness and disorder."[24] There is a range of medicalization, with spouse abuse being barely medicalized, menopause somewhat medicalized, and death, childbirth, and severe mental illness quite medicalized. Conrad noted that demedicalization occurs occasionally as well, as in the case of homosexuality being removed from the DSM. Conrad indicates that the direct marketing of mental illnesses as syndromes, covered by a wide range of medicines, has led to a reclassification of a variety of phenomena as mental illness, an expansion of medicalization.[25]

There are some instances of medicalization, such as the shift of epilepsy from mental illness to a neurological condition, that seem laudable. Others, such as the rise of major depression during a time of burgeoning inequity, seem more complex. Overmedicalization is a particular risk if poor persons and minorities get higher amounts of more powerful psychotropic drugs—that consequently have stronger side effects—when much of what they suffer from is caused by economic oppression. On the other hand, these marginalized groups are not given psychotherapy for their difficulties very often and thus the contribution of their own voice of explanation as to why they are suffering is diminished.[26]

The overmedicalization of mental distress is not neutral, but it is allied with certain power interests. In what follows I explain how the rise of biomedical psychiatry—with a diagnostic manual and an emphasis on pharmaceutical treatment—has lead to a disproportionate attention being placed on the supposed organic causes of mental illness to the diminishment of social and structural critique. This shift in emphasis has brought the disease entity to the fore while diminishing the social and structural factors that contribute to its course.

This shift in focus has the impact of blaming the victim by fostering individualistic cures for social problems. This does not take away the significance of individual interventions, but rather suggests that we have both misnamed the source and misappropriated resources to address suffering. By critiquing an exclusively biomedical approach, we do not diminish the impact that distress and emotional suffering have on the body and mind of a person-in-society. Rather, we refocus on the complex sources of meaning and interpretation that influence a person's view of the world and how these have been shaped specifically by economic suffering.

The current chapter explains why the contention that mental illness is a brain disease has been accepted by many ministers and counselors. I also provide a more contextual perspective through which to interpret mental illness. The payoff for this interpretive shift is that ministers and counselors can begin to resist the misattribution of suffering to the brain or genes of individuals when important social factors shape the course of this suffering. Once ministers make this shift, they can mobilize resources to better interpret and respond to the psychic suffering in their midst.

In the previous chapter we engaged extensively with the *epidemiology* of mental illness on a social scale, taking for granted concepts like anxiety, depression, or even schizophrenia, and then mapping them in relationship to different social factors such as debt or unemployment. Many of these studies used mental illness diagnostic categories from the International Classification or Diseases (ICD) or DSM. Such approaches can have the unintended effect of reifying the disease categories. In this chapter we explore how mental illness has been constructed as a disease concept, asking critical cultural and political questions about the promise and limits of this language. This is not for the sake of being deconstructionist, but rather to trace what has been missing in the medical model for mental illness.

The Rise of Biomedical Diagnostic Psychiatry

Emil Kraepelin, the predecessor to modern psychiatry, proposed that we could classify mental diseases according to a discrete set of symptoms categorized into a universal order.[27] In the late nineteenth century, he wrote index cards on each patient who entered the asylum and sorted these cards as he revised their diagnosis. He collected the results of his investigations into the *Lehrbuch fur Psychiatry* (1893), a volume that was published in several editions.

He intended to trace the inevitable progression of a disease rather than cure patients. Thinking that it was unnecessary to ask the patient about their emotional suffering—this could lead to error in the realm of research—he insisted that what was needed instead was a material basis for the science of mental illness. He saw patients as completely untrustworthy arbiters of the meanings of their disease, as he reported "we cannot afford to pay much attention to the patient's account of his experiences," and thus he neglected psychology entirely.[28] The story of the disease took center stage as the patient's story receded.

Reading symptoms meant reading the *reality* of the disease by naming it with scant attention to interpersonal experience. He presumed mental disease was rooted in disorders of the brain that lead to particular symptoms and hoped that science would eventually find the causes for these symptoms. Gary Greenberg summarizes, "by looking at what happened to the patient a doctor could judge with certainty the variety of madness that had been manifest in the patient's condition; the patient's fate would tell the doctor what disease he had in the first place."[29] This could be contrasted with germ theory that depended upon internal realities toward which symptoms of a disease referred.

Earlier in the nineteenth century, physicians had posited that some disorders were caused by endogenous factors—factors inside the person such as heredity or brain lesions—while others were caused from exogenous factors such as exposure to distressing stimuli. Kraepelin indicated that there were few if any cases of exogenous mental illness.[30] In the *descriptive turn* in psychiatry that Kraepelin proposed, if psychiatrists had an exhaustive list of diseases, they could have the "form of a science" that would discover the natural order of these diseases.[31] In a circular logic, "mental diseases...consisted only of lists of symptoms, and the symptoms were only symptoms because they belonged to the disease."[32] What mattered to Kraepelin was accurate diagnosis and this was a naming based on empirical observation. His opinion remained a minority view in his day.

Pharmacology

Kraepelin's point of view became more salient with the rise of compounds that were marketed for mental distress since these compounds came to be matched with particular disorders. Once the medicines were developed pharmaceutical companies sought a target—Kraepelin's descriptive psychiatry could provide one—at which to direct their compounds.

Understanding the story of biomedical psychiatry is impossible without describing the influence of pharmaceuticals. During the twentieth century, corporations began synthesizing derivatives of coal tar into medicines because of an excess in industrial products. In 1957 an over-the-counter sedative thalidomide was found to cause birth defects affecting as many as 6,000 children.[33] In 1962, the Food and Drug Administration decided that it needed "randomized, placebo-controlled, double-blind trials" in order to "establish the efficacy of a treatment" for each new medicine that would be prescribed.[34] In terms of research and development, corporations worked to make compounds that could be quite different from one another in their chemical effects but still be classed under the same category.

Psychopharmacology refers to the notion that studying the special effects of particular drugs on person's thinking and behavior will provide data for psychology, yet there is an absence of research in this field. For example, no tests could reliably demonstrate what drug someone has taken by noting changes in their behaviors. Early psychiatric drugs were marketed to endogenous illnesses, diseases that presumably stem from internal rather than external factors.

Throughout the history of psychotropic drugs, with the development of a new drug, disorders were described as the absence of that chemical.[35] In other words, people came to have disorders that were based on lacking the chemicals in their system that were developed and marketed by pharmaceutical corporations. Drugs can now be prescribed for a wide range of syndromes that are not major mental illnesses, and off-label use of pharmaceuticals is widespread, the conceptual reach of pharmacology has expanded.[36] Modern blockbusters such as Peter Kramer's *Listening to Prozac* invited people to read their experience back through the effects of antidepressants: "not infrequently...sufferers and their relatives confirm...the fact that they had not been so well for a long time," a telling description of this pharmacological approach.[37]

The theory of chemical imbalance in the brain was an overreach of scientific reasoning. Scientists isolated a compound that appeared to induce contractions in the gut wall and named it "serotonin," discovering that it could be found in the brain. This led researchers to suggest that nervous disorders may be the result of an *absence* of these chemicals in the brain, an inference that had no basis in brain research. Nevertheless, by taking a visual image of the pathways of serotonin through the brain and lighting it up with florescent lights, scientists gained wide acceptance for the idea that the brain worked by chemical transmission.[38] They argued for a time that these medicines were supposed to influence how serotonin was taken back up into the brain, but research has disproven this hypothesis.[39]

In other words, even before the antidepressant drugs were developed, scientists were busy working on explanations for how they could function. The ascendancy of biological research has provided a kind of "justification" and an appearance of "verisimilitude" for brain disease that has triumphed over other models of mental distress, in part because of the funding put into this research.[40]

Pharmaceutical explanations tend to exclude unfavorable data. For example corporations have downplayed the importance of the placebo effect— namely the significance of nonspecific factors such as the patient/ physician relationship that have a profound influence on "almost all psychiatric treatments."[41] Placebos performed as well as antidepressants in most trials.

Systemic research bias comes from corporate influence. Healy indicates that in the 1950s a group of corporations "sponsored the attendance of both clinical and preclinical investigators"[42] to research conferences and he underscores how "in the 1960s and 1970s an ever-greater proportion of scientists working in psychopharmacology or biological psychiatry were associated with the industry."[43] This finding has been corroborated in a series of recent research summarized by Marcia Angell, former editor of the *New England Journal of Medicine*.[44] Specifically, the pharmaceutical lobby suppresses research that challenges the effectiveness of its medicines, thereby promoting a selective view of pharmaceuticals. Now the theory of chemical imbalance in the brain has been thoroughly refuted,[45] antidepressants have been found to be less effective than earlier tricyclic drugs,[46] yet because the pharmaceutical industry suppresses studies that are critical of their drugs, it can be difficult to grasp such shifts.[47]

The discovery of certain mental illnesses seems to follow on the heels of the marketing of compounds by industry giants. Healy concludes, "It is clearly a mistake to think that mental illnesses are something that have an established reality and that the role of a drug company is to find the key that fits a predetermined lock."[48] In some cases, pharmaceutical companies seem able to keep a drug in the market despite serious side effects such as increased suicide risk, while other drugs, which have been deemed effective, have fallen out of favor because of bad press.[49]

Healy notes the "pharmacological Calvinism" of the United States, the belief that a drug is dangerous if it makes you feel good and that you will face some sort of "secular theological retribution" if you use it: "dependence, liver damage, chromosomal damage."[50] Some sectors of US society believe that medical approaches to psychic suffering represent a sign of weakness, such that "drug taking, even when officially sanctioned, remains an ambivalent reality in a culture that increasingly emphasizes the need for personal and interpersonal competence."[51] Because of pharmacological Calvinism there is a split between good and bad drugs. Some are approved by the government and marketed aggressively, while others presumably make you an addict and are warred upon.[52]

What we have in pharmacology is a reading of experience through the lens of drugs, but very little precise information about how the drugs work or, by extension, the mental illnesses that they purport to treat. In the case of depression, Healy maintains that it is not "a disorder of one neurotransmitter or a particular receptor but rather that in depressive disorders a number of physiological systems are compromised or... desynchronized in some way."[53] He speculates that "antidepressants" should have been sold over the counter as tonics rather than marketed as prescriptions for definable disorders.

In the pharmaceutical age there are a variety of competing explanations of mental illness based on divergent theories of how drugs function in the brain. An individual brain is typically the *subject* of such research, emphasizing what Dan Blazer calls a "methodological individualism."[54] In shorthand, this human person has a disease of the brain or genes that is epistemologically distinct from other diseases and thus can be categorized and thereby treated with medicine. In the remainder of the chapter we challenge this individual notion, proposing possible alternatives.

The aggressive marketing of compounds for discrete brain disorders paved the way for a return of endogenous psychiatry. As we saw earlier, Kraepelin proposed a descriptive framework that could explain mental illness but was pessimistic about the possibilities of treating it. With pharmaceuticals, a new era of descriptive nosology had begun without any of the pessimism.

The Return of Descriptive Psychiatry

In 1980, the American Psychiatric Association, under the leadership of Robert Spitzer, developed the third edition of the DSM, which was a bloodless coup against psychoanalytic and therapeutic models of psychiatry. The previous edition had used narrative prose that described neuroses and conflicts, but this version listed symptoms in an outline format. Whereas the second edition of the manual had 21 diagnoses and came in at 134 pages, this new version was 500 pages long. According to Spitzer, "the use of operational criteria for psychiatric diagnosis [was] an idea whose time [had] come."[55]

This list-of-symptoms approach to psychiatry presumes, like Kraepelin did, that organic or biological bases for mental illnesses exist that are yet to be found. Spitzer sought input from his colleagues about the kind of disorders they were treating and fashioned the volume specifically to make sure that insurance companies could reimburse for the medical treatment that was mental health care. Drug companies perceived an opportunity to link their medicines to specific disorders and syndromes, taking the invention of major depression for this purpose.[56]

The DSM-III was structured along several axes, the first of which is the major illness such as schizophrenia, bipolar, depression, or anxiety, and this was the necessary category for insurance reimbursement. The second axis is for personality disorders, what are seen as charactereological disorders such as borderline personality disorder. This category was unbillable on its own. The fourth axis described social factors such as life stressors that may have been a risk factor for the mental illness but was not seen as categorizing a mental illness in itself. Thus, no one can bill insurance because the factory has shut down, there are only nonunion service jobs, and the home is about to be foreclosed upon.

The language of scientific psychiatry, enshrined in Axis I diagnoses, is preeminent in the US medical and counseling system. Suddenly the diseases for which we have lacked the proper chemical balance, for example the absence of pharmaceutical drugs, are disorders in themselves. Although the latest edition of the DSM has abandoned the multiaxial system, in doing so they have emphasized the primacy of the biomedical model of mental illness. Now if there are Axis IV factors, they have to be placed in footnotes, indicating that there is an even larger gap that has been placed between mental illness and psychosocial stressors.[57]

What are the social factors that have contributed to this climate of opinion in which mental illness is largely seen as a brain disease? In a fascinating recent article about the invention of "major depression" as a clinical category, pastoral theologian Bruce Rogers-Vaughn argued that this development was closely linked to the phenomenon of neoliberalism, since in positing a biological origin of depression, the DSM reflects the emergence of a pharmaceutical industry that has gained increasing power. Simply giving persons medicine to make them happier seems to imply a vision of the individual who could be crafted into a more willing producer and consumer despite the fact that the real economic conditions surrounding the person (take-home income, access to quality housing) all deteriorating. He analyzes the consequences of this shift:

> Human misery is no longer due to any sociopolitical oppression, but is the responsibility of individuals themselves... they are simply unhappy because their brains are sick. Ultimately, this increases the suffering of depressed individuals... they only have themselves to blame and only they are responsible for getting themselves well again.[58]

According to Rogers-Vaughn, the rise of biomedical psychiatry itself is a political phenomenon. Healy summarizes, "the creation of a discrete set of disorders, such as panic disorder, social phobia, obsessive-compulsive, and other disorders gave the pharmaceutical industry a set of targets at which to aim its compounds" and this led to an internationalization and even an "American hegemony" of disease concepts.[59] As I noted, in the past several decades, if one relies upon medical insurance, one has had to be definably mentally ill, in categories drawn from the DSM's first axis, in order to be treated.[60] Even as the DSM abandoned its multiaxial model, it has lifted up Axis I, II, and III diagnoses and footnoted environmental and social factors. This heralds a new interpretive move in the history of human suffering: now the categories of diagnosis belong entirely with the medical psychiatrists.

Social Psychiatry and Psychiatric Auto-Critique

Let us briefly digress to explore an alternative to this descriptive approach. In the intervening years between the publication of Kraepelin's *Lehrbuch* (1893) and the DSM-III (1980), there were influential attempts to link mental distress to the social world. Swiss psychiatrist Adolf Meyer posited that a person's biography, particularly the life stresses they faced, were closely related to their experiences of suffering. Meyer was a key figure in what became known as social psychiatry.

This field studied "the effects of the social environment on the mental health of the individual, and... the effects of the mentally ill person on his or her own social environment."[61] According to Dan Blazer, social psychiatry was simultaneously an empirical science, a political movement, and a practice of mental health care in the community. Social psychiatry's research agenda focused on "the relationship between psychiatric disorders and the differences in populations and living conditions... understanding human motivation within the context of society... [and] how social organization... influences the definition of illness, the setting in which it arises, and provisions of care."[62] Meyer, for example, undertook detailed neighborhood studies to understand the social factors surrounding a child guidance clinic. Other researchers, such as Harry Stack Sullivan, used psychological research to address poverty, environmental destruction, and racism. These thinkers, some of whom were influenced by Frankfurt School Marxism, argued that the social conditions of modern life were untenable but that psychology ought to be used as one tool to transform these conditions. In what follows, I depict three influential psychiatrists, who, I argue, offer representative visions of social psychiatry.

Frantz Fanon was a psychiatrist from Martinique who was involved in liberation movements in Algiers, and whose work prefigured postcolonial thought. In his book *Black Skin, White Masks* he argued that understanding the oppression exhibited in colonial racism was crucial to understanding feelings of inferiority among black men. He analyzed dreams that included racial content and argued that culture promoted a valorization of whiteness that lead to psychic trauma for whites and blacks alike.

He noted that blacks only encountered feelings of inferiority upon entering Europe, indicating that these experiences were not the result of dysfunction or pathology, but a consequence of racism. For him, Jung's *collective unconscious* is fundamentally misguided in that it presumed that internal ideas could be inherited. Instead, "the collective unconscious is quite simply the repository of prejudices, myths, and collective attitudes of a particular group," for example, denigrating stereotypes about black male sexuality.[63] Addressing the situation for the colonial subject, he suggested that "any neurosis, any abnormal behavior... is the result of his cultural situation," since each person's mental problem was a combination of cultural oppression they had faced and the ways that they had responded to this oppression.[64] Critiquing a psychologist who described indigenous persons as having a "dependency complex," Fanon argued that "*it [was] the racist who create[d] the inferiorized.*"[65] Fanon stressed how a racist society diminished the humanity of the dominating and dominated alike and how it was impossible to understand issues like self-esteem and competition without interpreting the impact of structural racism. At the Blida asylum near Algiers, Fanon liberated patients from straightjackets and allowed them to smoke, encouraging his fellow psychiatrists to listen to them. When he helped these patients fight a revolution against the colonizers, one commentator wrote that "Freedom for the mad was a prelude to freedom for the colonized."[66]

In the United States, critiques of psychiatry have questioned the validity of mental illness as a diagnosis. In his 1961 text *The Myth of Mental Illness*, Thomas Szasz argued that hysterics were deemed to have an organic illness because Charcot, a powerful physician, received an implicit reward from this designation in terms of further authority and prestige. Exploring how Charcot's experiments were faked, Szasz indicated that the authority of the medical complex was at stake conceptually in the definition of mental illness as a neurological condition. The attribution of mental illness had a social-class component since "affluent psychiatric patients tend to receive psychotherapy, while poor patients were treated with physical interventions."[67] He was staunchly opposed to coercive psychiatry and the insanity defense and worked to make certain that he would never have to treat a coerced patient. At the same time, he supported psychotherapy as an ethical relationship between adults that needed to guard against the misuse of power. Szasz did not feel that mental illness could be treated more humanely without addressing the philosophical issues at play, namely the categorical mistake implied in the term: "Mental illness is a myth. Psychiatrists are not concerned with mental illnesses and their treatments. In actual practice they deal with personal, social, and ethical problems in living."[68] Late in life he summarized the heart of his critique, that "psychiatric power" has to do with the control of the bodies of others through forced hospitalization.[69] Unfortunately, his solutions were largely libertarian, which led to an excessive individualism. He appreciatively quoted Karl Popper, a philosopher who was involved in the development of neoliberalism, and suggested that each person could be said to be self-responsible, representing a radically contractarian position in psychiatry.

In 1955 Erich Fromm, a Marxist psychoanalyst, published *The Sane Society* in which he argued that we must not only diagnose the "adjustment" of individuals to a society but also "*the adjustment of society to the needs of man* [sic]."[70] His primary concern was a capitalist culture that had alienated persons from their labor. Referring to the assembly line worker, he notes that "his acts and their consequences have become his masters."[71] Arguing that the social situation of modern capitalism had commodified persons, he stated: "If the individual fails in a profitable investment of himself, he feels that *he* is a failure; if he succeeds, *he* is a success."[72] Describing the rise in suicides in industrial societies, he lamented how the individual worker had lost his or her role in the industrial process.[73]

Fromm suggested that advertising made us more insecure. He maintained, "our current psychiatric definitions of mental health stress those qualities which are part of the alienated social character of our time: adjustment, co-operativeness, aggressiveness...ambition, etc."[74] He maintained that it was impossible to offer an individualistic solution to the anomie that came from living in a capitalist society and instead advanced a form of communitarian socialism, advocating employee investment and decision making in corporate life, greater vacation time and work flexibility, and other work-based solutions that placed more autonomy into the lives of workers. In addition to advocating an ensured basic income, Fromm indicated that rehabilitating working conditions was crucial to improving the social circumstances of mental health. Writing during a time when greater prosperity occurred across US society, along with stronger union supports, it is striking that Fromm still noticed isolating aspects of capitalism and promoted a social psychiatry solution to them. In his language, it was primarily the alienated factory worker who suffered from meaninglessness—little did Fromm predict how globalization would change the face of manufacturing in the United States, leading many unemployed factory workers to long for aspects of the factory job.

With these theorists we are a long way from Peter Kramer's instant blockbuster *Listening to Prozac* that suggested we read our emotional lives through our experiences with pharmaceuticals, but instead it is necessary to listen to the holistic situation of the person in a culture with its social and economic arrangements. In the case of Frantz Fanon, Thomas Szasz, and Erich Fromm, we see efforts to integrate a more complex psychology that takes into account the various factors of modern existence. These authors creatively diagnose the dilemmas of our age and offer solutions that more holistically meet the psychic needs of persons.

In sum, many of the critics of psychiatry from within the discipline itself have offered trenchant critiques that continue to resonate. In the context of neoliberalism, what Fromm called "super-capitalism" has taken over,[75] with striking consequences for immigrants and minorities in the United States. In this context, the problems in living that persons face are more widespread, they are more closely linked to social conditions, and they require us to challenge the methodological individualism of an exclusively biomedical psychiatry. In passionate and direct language that addressed colonialism, Fanon expanded the critique of psychiatry by showing how the conditions of racial oppression directly contributed to emotional distress. Szasz critiqued psychiatric power's ability to coerce persons into a hospitalization because he did not believe the condition of mental illness was anything more than an exercise of medical authority. Finally, Fromm offered an image of a more just society and in the process placed the entire social system on the psychiatrist's couch.

In a time of runaway capitalism, people are more likely to diagnose themselves as failures if they do not make money. At the same, less resources are available to the working class to ameliorate this suffering, especially if they are African American or Latino/a. Understanding the social contexts of distress means proposing social solutions to our suffering, an approach that has been taken by critics within the discipline of psychiatry itself. In our discussion of the unique circumstances of our time, we draw on Szasz's profound skepticism, which necessitates a vision of the interdependent person-in-community as it is richly offered in Fanon and Fromm.

On the one hand social psychiatry consisted of thinkers like Fanon, Szasz, and Fromm, and on the other hand it was a public policy research agenda funded by the federal government that sought to improve the emotional welfare of the entire nation. This second kind of social psychiatry was about to change. At the end of the 1970s, more than half of the budget for the National Institute of Mental Health (NIMH) was devoted to researching social factors. In the 1980s Ronald Reagan came to power in the United States and stopped federal funding for community psychiatry, shifting the NIMH's budget to study biological origins of mental disorders rather than "social problems."[76] This shift matched trends in neoliberal thought toward personal responsibility and individual initiative. Taken together, this return to biomedical psychiatry represented the triumph of an earlier Kraepelinian model of mental disease, with the DSM-III (1980), and the subsequent rise of a psychopharmaceutical industry. Reagan's defunding legitimated a biomedical viewpoint by heavily subsidizing research that supported organic causes for mental illness while downplaying and even censoring social explorations that would have posited broad ranging solutions to social ills. In what follows, I explain how we are likely to attribute disorder to what is different, and how this diagnosis comes to redefine other aspects of a person's life.

Pathologizing Deviance: Gender and Race in Diagnosis

The conceit of descriptive psychiatry is that it objectively defines mental illness as existing in the brain of another, but evidence indicates that psychiatric judgments are historical and contingent, participating in complex ways with a bias. In his book *The Protest Psychosis: How Schizophrenia Became a Black Disease*, Jonathan Metzl studied the Ionia State Hospital for the Criminally Insane in Ionia, Michigan, and documented how the diagnosis of schizophrenia shifted over time. From the 1920s to the 1950s clinicians imagined that schizophrenics were primarily white women who suffered from emotional disharmony. Early pharmaceutical advertisements depicted white women working away at their sewing, presumably having been treated effectively for schizophrenia. The caption for this advertisement read "Clean, cooperative, and communicative."[77] This reflected a much longer history of pathologizing women.[78] In the nineteenth century, women were regularly committed to asylums against their will by their husbands, a practice that changed only with the advocacy of Elizabeth Parsons Ware Packard.[79] Yet, women continue to be diagnosed as pathological through hysteria, "histrionic personality disorder," and now "borderline personality disorder." According to the DSM-III, "hysterical personality" types were "overly dramatic and reactive...prone to exaggeration...often acting out the 'victim' or the 'princess' without being aware of it."[80] Such definitions represent sexist stereotypes under the guise of science. Deployed differently based on the gender of the psychiatrist who gives the diagnosis, it is clear that centuries-old constructions of gender persist in psychiatric nosology.[81]

With the reclassification of schizophrenia as a disease of black male aggression, "masculinized belligerence" in the second edition of the DSM in 1968, hundreds of black men were placed in the hospital and many were reclassified from having personality disorders to having major mental illness.[82] In the 1960s schizophrenia came to be seen as an illness that manifested rage, and black men were increasingly diagnosed with it. They were described as having "hostile and aggressive feelings" and "delusional anti-whiteness."[83] In pharmaceutical advertisements in the 1970s African American men were depicted in stereotypical terms and the medication was described as treating "hostile" and "belligerent" persons. In one advertisement for an antipsychotic, an African American man was depicted shaking his fist, a condition of aggression that was supposedly treated by pharmaceuticals. The advertisement stated, "cooperation begins with Haldol."[84]

For example, a man named Caesar Williams was held at Ionia State throughout the 1960s. On his first day at the hospital he hallucinated and threatened staff but was diagnosed with personality disturbance. Yet at the end of the decade his diagnosis was changed to paranoid schizophrenia despite the fact that "he had not changed during his hospitalization."[85]

As these offensive images show, within a few short years schizophrenia had a new face, indicating that a psychiatric diagnosis can shift in a very short period of time because of social conditions. Now race *and* social activism were construed together as pathogenic. The new form of schizophrenia suggested that "mental illness resulted not just from conditions of poverty, prejudice, and segregation, *but from political attempts to change them.*"[86]

Paradoxically, even the most progressive psychiatric treatments can reinforce stereotypes. In her anthropological exploration of three psychiatric hospitals in the New York City area that instituted a "Latino" program in the 1980s and 1990s through the Congress on Hispanic Mental Health (CHMH), Vilma Santiago-Irizarry describes how patients were constructed as having a particular Latino identity through a hospital program, and how culture was positioned as something that had to be overcome by treatment. Strangely, it was assumed that culture could heal, but patients were also expected to progress beyond culture.

On these "Latino" wings of the hospital, the staff spoke Spanish, served traditionally "ethnic" foods, and decorated the wards based on a supposedly homogenous Latin culture. This constructed pan-Latino identity came to take the place of more rights-based activities such as translating medication forms into Spanish, since such activities did not seem "ethnic" enough.[87] From the beginning, the project was fraught with difficulties since none of the patients seemed to know what it meant to be on a "cultural" ward.[88] This "Latino" program was imposed upon patients from several continents who spoke in various Spanish dialects, who occupied different generations and immigration statuses, and who were from different social classes.

Within this conception of a "cultural" wing, while speaking Spanish was supposed to help patients improve, speaking Spanish was also a site of regression from psychological health. On the one hand, "the abreaction of the self is so prized in mental health care. Patients were expected to 'open' their selves through talk to staff."[89] On the other hand, the Spanish language was perceived as a hindrance and part of a person's sickness. When patients reverted to Spanish, a Latino psychiatrist claimed, "[the psyche] [was] divested of its socialization and return[ed] to a 'raw' state of psychic fragmentation."[90] Likewise, a one-dimensional view of language emerged: the program constructed patients' language capacities as "bilingual" rather than as a mixture of code switching and accents.

She indicated that this project of ethnicizing patients was a complicated veiling of economic oppression. While a third of Latinos lived in poverty they had been positioned as *deserving* poverty through a pan-Latino identity. Santiago-Irizzary cites the US research on "Special Populations" in the 1970s that stated that "Hispanics subsist in a 'culture of poverty'... they are superstitious, unacculturated, and have clearly defined and retrogressive structures and roles."[91] Through this offensive language, Latinos are implicitly blamed for living in poverty even as they are constructed as a special group with a universal identity that must be overcome on the way to assimilation.

As we have seen, projects that attempt to provide cross-cultural care can often construct culture as an obstacle on the way to the "health," where health here is the presumed normativity of a dominating cultural group. Something similar happens across the psychiatric literature, and texts in pastoral care and counseling as well, when there is a small section in a text on the problem of cultural awareness or when ethnicity is described in essentialized features that may cover over linguistic specificity, social location, language status, and other factors.[92] When this happens, the discourse of the "psy-complex," the various disciplines of psychiatry, psychology, and social work, as well as the institutional settings in which they are deployed,[93] can seem universal. The psy-complex is thus healthy while the "ethnic" is described as that which has to be overcome. What becomes clear is that psychiatric discourse's power can be put into place in particular institutional settings where it relies both on what is said and what remains unsaid by positioning others as "contextual" while at the same time obscuring its own contextual nature.

The social frame indelibly marks the clinical encounter. It is impossible to separate the power of diagnosis from a close and critical reading of culture, because rapid shifts in social life create radically different diagnoses. Becoming more culturally competent is not enough unless one examines fundamental structures such as sexism and racism that impact the diagnostic process. The normative force of psychiatry is shaped by the exclusion of difference and this exclusion is reinforced through diagnosis.

The implication here is that a social and structural analysis of pervasive factors such as racism, sexism, classism, and heterosexism does not belong as an add-on to psychiatry, but instead is an indispensable prerequisite. At the same time, structural analysis must be used in a continual way to critique the clinical frame's presumption to know what it "sees" in front of it. This is important because the diagnosis of mental illness—including the language used in such diagnosis—does not exist in a vacuum but is operationalized in particular institutional spaces.

It is one thing to acknowledge that culture and context impact the clinical frame, but it is important to note precisely how they do so and that this impact can be assessed in the psychiatrist/patient relationship. The DSM-III in 1980 was supposedly more reliable, having been field tested, but a study in 1988 indicated that psychiatrists using this version were biased based on perceived gender and race. Although the findings are complex, they are worth reviewing in some detail here. The experiment was tested on patients who were black men, black women, white men, and white women. Likewise, the psychiatrists were variously black men, black women, white men, and white women. The experiment involved sending two case studies to a group of psychiatrists that included reports of trouble sleeping, seeing visions, and unemployment.

When the race and gender of the client were not attached to the study, most psychiatrists diagnosed the patient with "undifferentiated schizophrenic disorder," the milder of the conditions rather than "paranoid schizophrenia," which consisted of "prominent persecutory or grandiose delusions, or hallucinations with a persecutory or grandiose content... including unfocused anxiety, anger, argumentativeness, and violence."[94]

The researchers found that black psychiatrists, both male and female, gave the white males the least serious diagnosis (undifferentiated schizophrenic disorder), while white females gave white males the more serious diagnosis (paranoid schizophrenia). None of the white male psychiatrists gave a white male patient the diagnosis of paranoid schizophrenia and black males were more likely than any other group to be deemed paranoid schizophrenic.

Some of the psychiatrists were given *no* information about race and gender and many of them were dissatisfied in making a diagnosis without these contextual markers. Nineteen refused to fill in the diagnostic categories because they felt they did not have enough information about the clients.

The patient's social location *and* the psychiatrist's social location are both significant in the perception of illness. Diagnosis occurs in the context of a particular relationship and cultural setting but with a marked power differential between the two parties. Indeed, rather than offering universalizable properties that apply evenly in all circumstances, diagnostic frames interact in complex ways with the people who have the power to diagnose. There is no direct match between the body and brain of the ill and the expert's diagnostic categories, but invariably the psychiatrist's perceptual framework impacts their diagnostic practices.

This perception of difference can have lasting effects. Metzl described how, after deinstitutionalization, the men in Michigan were still held in the mental hospital through a loophole for those who were deemed dangerous to the community. At the end of the 1970s, the mental hospital changed into a prison, the Riverside Correctional Facility, but the floor plan of the institution did not change and many of the patients continued to be held. These mental patients were now reclassified as inmates and deemed dangerous. This pattern continues today, when there are more people diagnosed with schizophrenia in prisons than in psychiatric hospitals.[95]

Deinstitutionalization and Managed Care

Vast social changes have happened in the last several decades that have stripped mental health support from the communities that need it most. While such care may need to be reformed so that it does not pathologize deviance, we also need a much broader safety net of financial and social supports to help struggling persons. The infrastructure of support has been dismantled.

In 1963 President Kennedy set forth the Community Mental Health Act, an ambitious new program that hoped to reform state mental institutions by establishing community centers for mental health, but this program was inadequately funded because of the Vietnam War and the economic downturn. In 1965 Medicaid incentivized communities to move mentally ill patients into nursing homes. Although Jimmy Carter in 1980 proposed a new program to fund community mental health, the very next year it was defunded by Reagan who decreased mental health spending by a third. The result of this process has been "deinstitutionalization," a "set of policies and treatment innovations that drove the more than half-million person decrease in the population of state and county mental hospitals between 1965 and the present."[96] "In 1955... 559,000 persons were institutionalized in state mental hospitals out of a total net population of 165 million. Now the figure is 72,000 for a population of more than 250 million."[97] Where have these people gone?

Transinstitutionalization refers to the movement from mental hospitals to jails and prisons. In the definitive work on the subject Raphael and Stoll maintain that "a sizable portion of the mentally ill behind bars today would not have been incarcerated in years past."[98] As I noted earlier, more schizophrenics are in prison than in mental hospitals today. The author's research lead them to conclude that "this highly statistically significant estimate for white males suggests a near one-for-one transfer rate from mental hospitals to prisons over this time period. For black males, the estimate suggests a one-half-for-one transfer rate" with much lower percentages for women, Hispanics, and people of other ethnicities.[99] The mentally ill were more likely to be serving for a property crime than violent crimes or drug offenses, and more than 17 percent were homeless before arrest, as compared with six percent in the general population.[100]

It seems that many people who had been in mental hospitals end up on the streets. Deinstitutionalization has been a lengthy process beginning in the 1940s and 1950s, but in the early years patients received more support and were thus less likely to become homeless. According to a Housing and Urban Development, 26 percent of the homeless had severe mental illness.[101] During the 1980s, the help given to the mentally ill had changed from hospitals to disability payments and persons who were mentally ill were offered treatment for their disease, but with little help or subsistence. While deinstitutionalization promised to shift money to communities to pay for resources, the money saved by closing state hospitals was seldom redistributed to the states to pay for mental health care as promised. As a result, the care systems were often ill equipped to provide the kind of multidimensional support (work, housing) that was needed for persons experiencing mental distress.[102]

While support for those with more severe forms of mental distress has shrunk, so has support for people with everyday problems in living. With the advent of health maintenance organizations (HMOs) and managed care during the 1990s, mental health came to be performance-monitored. Only people who had "medical necessity" could be treated.[103] Under managed care people are assessed based upon their level of functioning, which is then addressed with short-term behavioral approaches that attempt to return them as quickly as possible to higher levels of functioning.[104] Although the Global Assessment of Functioning (GAF) has been replaced in the most recent edition of the DSM, there is still a functional approach enshrined in this medical model of mental illness, which places categorizable mental illness first and subsumes all social and environmental factors to footnotes. With disorder in the forefront, counseling and care become increasingly the province of biomedical psychiatry. Because managed care has profoundly impacted how people in the United States utilize mental health services, this rise in functionalism, with the resulting diminishment of an emphasis on the social world, has culminated in quantification at the expense of addressing the root factors contributing to mental distress. The manner in which deinstitutionalization has taken place in the states, combined with the shrinking of mental health services into a managed care framework, suggests that there is less and less space to tell complex narratives about the causes, course, and consequences of our problems in living.

All of these changes refer to the shifts that have occurred in the neoliberal era in the United States. Deinstitutionalization was both idealistic and pragmatic at the same time and it fit into the logic of neoliberalism by shifting responsibility for mental suffering to individuals.[105] As we have seen, neoliberalism promotes freeing private enterprise and making the individual responsible for their well-being. According to this limited conception, each person has adequate resources to advocate for the best mental health treatment for themselves and their families, emphasizing everyone's private choice. Yet the struggles that face the mentally distressed are many, and these cannot be adequately captured in managed care's functionalist approach. When resources to help the homeless mentally ill are absent, and dominant themes from the media and self-help books reemphasize an ethic of individual initiative and autonomy, little wonder people turn inward to blame themselves for their problems in living. All too often, people see themselves as failures rather than critiquing the failure of the promised American Dream.

This leads to an important set of questions that are in the background of social science research on economics and mental illness. Are people diagnosed with mental disorders *because* of the stress that accompanies poverty or does being perceived as poor *lead* to the diagnoses of mental illness? While it may not be possible to completely answer this question, its implications are important. If the first approach is taken, it could lead to practical alleviation of the circumstances that contribute to poverty but the power exerted through the diagnostic frame would be left largely intact. If the second approach is taken, a strong critique of psychiatric power could emerge, but the class aspects of disempowerment that attend the experience of being made poor would be less clearly articulated. Neither approach is ultimately satisfactory in themselves.

Thankfully we do not have to make a false choice. In his book *Pastoral Care and Liberation Theology,* Stephen Pattison gestures toward a model for integration. On the one hand, "there appear to be factors within our present capitalist social order which lead to a greater incidence and prevalence of identified mental illness amongst working-class people."[106] In other words, society creates conditions that lead to extreme distress. On the other hand, he also refers to a more discomforting reality that is seen often in the sociological literature about mental illness: "People from the lowest social classes 'enjoy' a higher rate of diagnosis of clinical mental disorder."[107] Impoverished people are more likely to be diagnosed as mentally ill.

This was seen in the "culture of poverty" discourse used against the Puerto Rican patients in the New York hospital system.[108] To describe the suffering caused by poverty in exclusively individualistic terms contributes to blaming those who are made poor for their predicament. In each instance that we attempt to address social suffering, we must be careful of the discourse that we use to describe it lest we contribute to this phenomenon.

Nevertheless, the suffering that comes from economic injustice is real and must be named in some manner. Understanding how economic conditions contribute to psychological discourse is one step. A concurrent step is to critique how psychiatry helps reinforce notions that poverty is somehow one's fault, as through the "culture of poverty" discourse in its variations. This is especially important because the mistaken culture of poverty discourse has contributed to the stripping away of social safety nets by Democrats and Republicans alike. Understanding the consequences of oppression means exploring the economic and political factors that lead to social distress and economic disenfranchisement.

Conceptualizing Suffering

Mental health professionals and religious leaders have a significant role to play in helping people interpret their suffering. Counselors are likely to use functionalist categories of mental health to justify insurance reimbursement, but they are also free to interpret how social factors may be impacting peoples' lives. Ministers often have an opportunity to travel with people and their communities over a long period of time, and they may be privileged to hear the unique questions facing persons affected by economic distress: "Why is God letting this happen to me?" and "Am I crazy?"

If psychiatric power consists in a methodological individualism that roots mental suffering in the brain and genes of a person, there is room for a wider imagination that sees how people are shaped by complex social forces.

Understanding how mental illness refers to person's problems in living but is also a social construct that encompasses deviance, a minister can imagine a person as more than a diagnosis that needs to be treated with medication. Rather, envisioning the entire-person-in-context, one can exercise a pastoral imagination that sees the real extent of social suffering brought about by oppression and how this has an impact on the minds and bodies of individuals in communities.

A family that has been going through a difficult time—the father seems about to lose his job—and is also going through the psychiatric hospitalization of its eldest child, comes in and sits down in the minister's office. The father asks the minister, "Am I going crazy?" The mother states, "I don't believe my daughter has a mental illness. What do you think?" The minister looks at the family altogether and says: "I think you have a dysfunctional family."

Given the research presented in chapters 1 and 2, this pastoral scenario needs to be re-imagined, not treating this family as simply "imbalanced" in some way, or lacking some necessary chemical in their minds. Likewise, the entire social context of their suffering needs to be addressed. A minister may have posters discussing economic inequity on her wall or over her desk, indicating that she understands the broader economic context in which they operate. At the same time, it may be helpful to simply ask a provocative question, "What if it isn't something wrong with you? What if it's the wider society in which we live?"[109]

Ministers and counselors are faced with epistemological questions—questions about the status of knowledge—in their work everyday. In grappling with these epistemological questions they are grappling with theological anthropology, asking questions about what it means to be a human created in the image of God with unique gifts and inalienable dignity.

Many ministers already understand the social factors bearing down on people because they are going through similar stresses themselves. Counselors, however, especially those responsible for psychiatric diagnosis, have a trickier job. They have to grapple with the socially constructed labels that they must use to describe human suffering while engaging in self-critical analysis of the discourse that they use and the context in which they are deployed. In each case, ministers and pastoral counselors do their best to provide whatever can be used to alleviate suffering while resisting, at the same time, the idea that the suffering is exclusively caused from inside the person.

With this evidence before us there are a range of interpretive options. Some readers could wonder whether the epistemological framework of psychiatry is sound and what needs to be replaced are merely the sexist, racist, and classist frameworks that filter its data. These readers might describe the research noted previously as consisting of the poor practice of a medical science that is still valid. Others may have questions that are equally profound—what about people who experience their mental illness diagnosis as a helpful clarification of important aspects of their lives? Does such research require rejecting biomedical explanations entirely? Given the widespread nature of human suffering and its causes, an objection might be that we simply use psychiatric discourse *as it is* to help address this suffering, for example the widespread links between poverty and various mental illnesses described in the previous chapter.

Rather than offer another critique of psychiatry, why not advocate for better treatment? There are a range of approaches possible here as well: reducing the criminalization of those diagnosed with mental illness and finding housing for them, their forced confessions to crimes not committed, and their execution for these crimes in the United States. As we have seen in the neoliberal era there is also the lack of access to mental health care, especially for people in the working class. There is a real form of suffering that is faced by people in the new economy: simply redefining it as an effect of power will not be adequate to address this suffering.

At the same time we must grapple with the effects of psychiatric power in order to be honest. If we are not clear about the corporate and conceptual interests behind the terms we use, we risk turning these terms into concrete realities by imbuing them with an epistemological priority that is unsound.

All helpful medical, therapeutic, and religious interventions should be used to help people suffering in this new economy. We should not slip into our own pharmacological Calvinism and expect people suffering in the new economy to be able to "pull themselves up by their bootstraps." All means of relieving suffering is necessary, but caution should be exerted lest people feel that their identity is derived from a mental health perspective only, especially when the experience of suffering is so deeply crafted by the social world.

The field of pastoral care and counseling borrows many of its presumptions from the field of psychiatry and for this reason the overmedicalization of psychiatry has led to pastoral care foregoing important social explanations for mental illness and reducing the human person to the brain and genes. Within a psychiatric framework the Axis I diagnosis have primacy while social factors move to the footnotes, frequently to be addressed by social workers, ministers, or nurses. The consequences of this shift is that which is primary gets confused. What should be seen as symptoms of social suffering—anxiety, distress, discouragement all due to the impending home foreclosure—are placed in the background while a presumably universal disease process comes to the foreground to take up the clinician's attention. This is a political concern because important misunderstandings can occur when our attention is diverted in this fashion.

Using mental health categories exclusively to diagnose emotional problems when the stress from the social world impinges upon a person seems inadequate. I described in the introduction the tendency of the psy-complex to methodological individualism. With the advent of psychopharmacology, there were pills that people could take for anxiety and depression, but the implication of taking these pills is that a person is sick rather than oppressed. At the same time, a powerful organizational lobby had an interest in promoting these drugs and the disorders they presumed to treat, including new disorders such as social phobia and attention-deficit disorder, and this lobbying led to widespread expansion of the notion of mental illness from a biomedical perspective.

The social suffering of our neoliberal era can make us sick but we should refuse individualistic labels for the illness from which we suffer.[110] In other words we should challenge the reductionism inherent in psychiatric naming even as we attempt to address the psychic suffering that people face.

We are missing some significant aspects of the emotional suffering of our current times and its tone if we rely on biomedical models of mental illness only. We tend to evaluate ourselves based on the images that we are incited to consume, including images that advertise treatments for our psychopathology and its causes rather than problems rooted in the social sphere. Biomedical psychiatry as an exclusive explanation of mental illness plays into the themes of neoliberalism by emphasizing a person who is meant to be an entrepreneur of themselves, pulling themselves up by their bootstraps. All too often this has the effect of helping people adjust to circumstances rather than addressing these circumstances directly. People are incited to measure themselves and they come up wanting. They frequently attempt to refill what is lacking through medical means, by adjusting the chemicals in their brains, when they also need an opportunity to address the root causes of this suffering.

In the next chapter I describe consumer/survivor/ex-patient (c/s/x) activism as a challenge to psychiatric power. One significant aspect of the c/s/x approach is being able to name for oneself one's own values and preferences in the face of what can become an all-encompassing identity. C/s/x activism tends to be more radical than simply educating about the symptoms of mental illness in order to diminish stigma. It involves analyzing the power that is used in the psychiatric relationship itself. As we see in this chapter, such analysis must be multidimensional and include a critique of the psychiatric system of diagnosis, its roots in phychopharmacology, as well as a critique of the social-class system that places undue suffering on certain individuals. Expanding ministerial imagination means seeing people as more than simply disordered brains or genes, but foregrounding the social suffering stemming from the world in which they live.

CHAPTER 3

In Their Own Words: Mental Health Consumers, Survivors, and Ex-Patients

In chapters 1 and 2 of this book, I described the extent to which economic suffering was contributing to mental distress and how biomedical psychiatry alone did not account adequately for the kind of suffering that was so often social in nature. I described some psychiatric critics who challenged the biomedical framework, but in this chapter I argue that we must move beyond expert voices. This chapter explores some representative ways that people who have been involved with the mental health system interpret their distress.

It is necessary to attend to the voices of those most impacted by mental illness diagnoses, including how they name their own experiences, for example, distress, exultation. We might call this a *preferential option for the most silenced stories*. This chapter links themes of self-definition with self-determination. Self-definition is the ability to name one's own experience and to choose what matters most. Self-determination is linked to a host of other macro-factors such as housing, material goods, and social welfare and it provides the basis for self-definition.

In this chapter, I discuss some of the primary literature in the field of consumer/survivor/ex-patient movements. Rather than the narratives of family members—an important subject in its own right—the narratives of psychiatrized persons are discussed in this chapter. Concepts such as a disease model for mental illness will not be critiqued in this chapter, but neither will it be endorsed.[1] If discourse used in psychiatric spaces emphasize the physician's words about the patient, alternative approaches foreground activist's voices and concerns.

Based on the activism and advocacy work of a group sometimes called consumer/survivor/ex-patients, this chapter explores the various positions from which activism originates: "mental health consumers" who engage in activism while using mental health services to some extent, "survivors" who tend to reject these services altogether, and "ex-patients" who emphasize their own skills for recovery from mental suffering, noting how they have exited the patient role.[2] It is important to note that the c/s/x movement contains a *range* of positions toward the conceptual status of mental illness and also a range for engaging with treatments endorsed by medical science. This chapter also analyzes the c/s/x movement in light of social-class theory, arguing that directly addressing economic factors is an important emerging concern for the c/s/x movement.

In this chapter I explore the epistemological perspectives of c/s/x activists. Epistemology refers the status of knowledge and the implications of knowledge. C/s/x activism is rooted in a complex intellectual heritage drawn from phenomenology, sociology, and ethnomethodology, and the struggles of working-class rights, as well as feminism, LGBTQ rights, and civil rights. C/s/x advocacy often coalesces around the problematic aspects of psychiatric power, seeking to reclaim some power for activists in the movement. This can be done through interventions such psychiatric advanced directives in which people have a chance to articulate their preference for psychiatric treatment, informed consent about psychiatric medications' side effects, forced hospitalization, and other foci such as housing, employment, and discrimination.

Given the information about transinstitutionalization (the movement from mental hospital to prison) laid out in the previous chapter, it is necessary to read c/s/x activism in conversation with a broad human rights agenda. As we have seen, once persons were deinstitutionalized they entered communities that were not very welcoming of their difference, leading to transinstitutionalization in prisons. Addressing such basic self-determination concerns against the backdrop of a neoliberal economy means providing housing, food, and clothing within an environment of care so that a person's voice can be heard. This should be done in user-oriented spaces where themes of coping, recovery, and peer-support come to the fore, rather than clinical spaces that reinforce a fixed identity as a mental patient.[3] Since emotional distress affects more people than ever in a neoliberal economy, making these support-structure changes is essential to the well-being of the entire society.

In my analysis of these resources, I focus on the interpretive and meaning-making tools of c/s/x activism and how these tools are both similar to and different from Marxist analysis of working-class positions and disability studies that focus on intellectual disability. The fundamental focus of this chapter is on hearing the stories of those diagnosed with mental illness and how this is a crucial aspect of fostering their own dignity. My hope is that ministers and pastoral counselors will learn to advocate for people diagnosed with mental illness through fostering concrete realities such as housing support, as well as helping them at the level of discourse by hearing their voices and self-definition. This can be done by facilitating peer support in their communities.

On Our Own: The First Mental Health User Memoir

In 1971, the first mental health advocacy organization formed in New York—the Mental Patients Liberation Project. One of the original leading spokespersons was Judi Chamberlin. She published a moving memoir in 1978—*On Our Own: Patient-Controlled Alternatives to the Mental Health System*—that included well-researched argumentation for user-facilitated services. Here she set forward a bill of rights for mental patients that was based on the fundamental dignity of the human, the right to informed consent for medication and treatment, legal and medical counsel, "uncensored communication," the right to bring grievances, the right to be notified before being used in medical tests, and the right to refuse hospitalization in favor of an alternative to the mental health system.[4] This early language of rights, rooted in the mad liberation movement, paved the way for future organizing around specific rights-based issues in the 1990s.

Chamberlin's memoir describes her experiences in mental hospitals, where she reported being ignored, not told where she was being taken, and having the doors locked to keep her inside. She offers one telling piece of conversation with her doctor. In this conversation her doctor was arguing for her being placed in a state hospital rather than the private one where she was staying:

"Why can't I stay here?"
"This isn't a long-term hospital. You need long-term care."
"Let me go home. I'll go back to my psychiatrist. I'll see him every day."
"You're too sick to go home."
"But a state hospital—they don't give any care there. Let me go someplace where I can get treatment."
"You don't need treatment. You need long-term custodial care."

"What's wrong with me? What's the name of it?"
"You have a character disorder. You need to be in a place with a rigid structure. You may never be able to live outside a hospital."[5]

In this interchange Chamberlin and her doctor engage in an unbalanced discourse in which she tries to negotiate her circumstances within the doctor's realm of the mental hospital. Chamberlin emphasizes the tremendous power differential that exists between mental health patients and professionals in the field of psychiatry, and she argues for patient-controlled alternatives to the current mental health system.

Along with the power invested in the management of psychiatric patients, there is also an everyday power that constructs the mentally ill as an identity differing from the norm. Chamberlin coins the term mentalism that she defines as conscious or unconscious prejudice against people with emotional distress by the outside society or by persons who have been diagnosed.

> Like racism and sexism, mentalism infects its victims with the belief in their own inferiority, which must be consciously rooted out. By working together in self-help organizations, ex-patients can gain experience in helping themselves and one another. But the belief in one's own inferiority can continue unless active efforts are made to combat it.[6]

The flip side of mentalism has been described as "sanism," which is a conscious or unconscious phobia of people suffering from emotional distress that asserts itself a need to confirm one's own sanity and normalcy. Sanism is often based on the ideal of the "normate," or "the social figure through which people can represent themselves as definitive human beings."[7] Mentalism interacts with other forms of oppression such as gender, racial, and social-class discrimination to lead to multiple levels of marginalization.[8]

Significantly, she includes social class as a category in this power imbalance: "Psychiatrists (who are often middle or upper class) may never have faced the kinds of problems their poorer patients face daily," and she notes that the problems of living faced by poor people seldom become the focus of psychiatric treatment.[9] Mentalism interacts with other forms of oppression but is not reducible to them. Although the ability to see her psychiatrist everyday indicates that she belonged to the owner class, Chamberlin's class position still did not win her any more power in the psychiatrist–patient interaction.

For example, Chamberlin contrasts the demeaning interaction that she had with her psychiatrist with the interaction with her peers. She met a friendly patient named Harry who helped her interpret her skin crawling and stomach churning: "When I told him what I had been taking, he understood. 'You're having withdrawal symptoms.'"[10] This interchange highlights the significance of peer support for mental health difficulties. No one among the medical staff had bothered to warn her of withdrawal symptoms when they took her off a powerful drug. Whereas the power imbalance in the psychiatrist's speech was obvious, the friendliness of another patient provided tremendous relief to Chamberlin and also contributed to clarity about her situation.

As we saw in the previous chapter, discourse is the power to name and the contexts which endorse such naming, and official speech can be distinguished from peer-oriented speech. Discourse about mental illness shared in peer support spaces tends to draw from everyday terminology and resist the attribution of pathology. Unofficial speech between patients is a different context for discourse than professional speech. Understanding discourse in this way helps us grasp the differences in clinical and peer-centered speech in a variety of contexts.[11]

Chamberlin argues that patients should develop their own groups in which they provide support for one another through emotional difficulties. In her view, these would be "voluntary, small, and responsive to their own communities."[12] On a practical level, Chamberlin argues that people who have "difficulties in living" are frequently able to help one another—"Being able to reach out to another person—even when one is feeling bad oneself—illustrates to the person in distress that he or she is not incompetent or worthless."[13] For Chamberlin what is at stake is the dignity of self-determination in daily decisions, such as the freedom to come and go and choose what one wants for dinner. She gives an example of how she was helped through an acute psychiatric episode by a fellow c/s/x activist in a peer-run support center, indicating that shared experience and accompaniment were the key factors necessary for mental health recovery in peer-run settings.

She argues that the primary issue in the psychiatric system is power. Indicating that such power is based on a problematic assertion of power, she names the rights issues at stake. The fundamental conceptual mistake of reading psychiatric behaviors as symptoms analogous to the symptoms of a physical disease, combined with the exaggeration of the dangerousness of mental patients, has led to a situation where the rights of people deemed mentally ill have been systematically eroded. "The law has the power to compel people to receive treatment for mental illness," she states, through a comparison of the mental patient to a child.[14]

Through analysis of her experience, Chamberlin described elements of valid psychiatric alternatives, including the needs of the service institution being defined by the clients, voluntary participation in all or some of the services, placing responsibility for financial decisions in client hands, peer-run and selected services, and client control over information. This approach promises to be holistic and egalitarian, so that "the ability to give help is seen as a human attribute and not as something acquired by education or professional degree."[15] At the heart of her project is a challenge to the sense of profound helplessness and lack of control that many people associate with the idea of mental illness. Instead, there is a foregrounding of the person who is able to determine what is important to them. In Chamberlin's book we read of an ethical humanism that informs organizing, including a deep respect for the experience of the other. In her estimation, the person suffering from mental distress is an agent with full dignity.

Many of the books in pastoral care and counseling on the subject of mental illness focus on families. Other books focus on congregations becoming more welcoming. Recent approaches focus topically on different forms of mental illness. The few texts that focus on the experience of people diagnosed with mental illness and their ability to voice their own perspectives, tend to use clinical categories drawn from the DSM as primary descriptors.[16] Yet there are several user-based perspectives that frequently are neglected in the clinical frame.

Self-recovery movements have been an underexplored theme in pastoral care. People who hear voices are beginning to define their own experience of this phenomenon, and ministers and counselors benefit from hearing their self-definition. Chamberlin's work underscores the conceptual difficulties we encounter in placing the stories of c/s/x activists first, rather than privileging a professional perspective about mental illness.

Themes and Controversies in the C/S/X Movement

In what follows, I describe Mad Liberation, which is the civil rights movement on which the mental patients' liberation movement is based, and then I describe each of the conceptual turns of the movement. In *Talking Back to Psychiatry: The Psychiatric Consumer/Survivor/Ex-Patient Movement*, Linda Morrison interviewed advocates at the grassroots level who were involved in community organizing and rights work and gave a conceptual history of the c/s/x movement. She identified the principles at the heart of the movement: people must have a voice in their treatment, access to legal rights, protection from harm, "the power of self-determination," and "choice in their treatment and their lives."[17] In what follows, we describe the liberation movement that undergirds such activism and we analyze the survivor, consumer, and ex-patient categories in turn.

Mad Liberation

The movement to liberate persons from mental "treatment" began with movements such as feminist, antiracist, and gay and lesbian liberation. Phyllis Chesler's significant early work *Women and Madness* indicates that feminism was important to the mad liberation movement. Indeed, she links psychiatry with patriarchy and offers a conceptual basis for critiquing both.[18] Similarly, Chamberlin cited the importance of feminism as an influence that helped her leave her first marriage, which she described as contributing to her mental difficulties.

An early forum for the c/s/x liberation movement was *Madness Network News* (MNN), a San Francisco–based publication that brought together critical mental health professionals and survivors who, under the rubric of "Breaking the Silence," sought to expose "the 'knots'/Catch 22's/ mind catch of the psychiatric system."[19]

From the beginning mad liberation was linked with class activism. The first edition of MNN was sponsored by the Social Service Employee's Union and linked the "voices of... psychiatrized persons and workers."[20] From its inception, mad liberation movement was funded by unions and included working-class themes. This is worth emphasizing because it is a seldom-acknowledged reality about the mad liberation movement. The connection to labor issues made it more likely that people would connect the dots between economic and psychiatric oppression. Indeed, the early activists speaking at the 1975 Conference on Human Rights and Psychiatric Oppression described "suffering as a result of social conditions rather than mental illness."[21] Working-class concerns were linked explicitly to the concerns of mental patients who were seen as marginalized in the economic order.

Voice was a contentious issue from the movement's inception. Who would be considered an author[ity] in the movement? While MNN initially contained readings from Szasz and Foucault, later editions shifted to survivor testimonies. Leaders of the movement included Judy Chamberlin, Howie the Harp, Sally Zinman, Leonard Roy Frank, Su Budd, Jay Mahler, David Oaks, Janet Foner, and Joseph Rogers. Although there was a range of positions on controversial issues such as medication even in the early movement, there was an overarching concern about self-determination and voice. What these themes invariably combined was "advocacy and mutual support."[22]

On the advocacy side, civil liberties concerns about being confined against one's will, experiencing shock treatments, being experimented upon without one's consent, all provided the primary content for advocacy. A telling example of the importance of advocacy comes from the history of mad liberation itself. At a 1975 mad liberation conference, c/s/x activists noted that suddenly the entire control of the meeting had been wrested from them, with professionals speaking for them and all the conference meetings being run by educators and psychiatrists. Now c/s/x advocates were placed in a precarious position: the very conference they began had been organized away from them. So they protested outside the doors, demanding to have their voice heard by professionals who had imposed their own perspectives.[23]

Advocacy had to do with some level of resistance to discourse, the offering of alternative languages to describe mental illness, and dignifying experiences that were different from the norm. Identity politics coalesced around key psychiatric concerns such as coercion, shock treatment, and forced hospitalization, while at the same time the conceptual categories of psychiatry were called into question. Advocacy was supplemented by more representational and meaning-making tasks such as writing poetry or creating art that defined one's own experience of mental distress.

On the mutual support side, early mad liberation sought to offer practical alternatives for the care of persons suffering from emotional distress. Echoing Chamberlin, on the self-help side it was clear that "people did have emotional and other life problems that they needed some place to go to for help and support" so client-run alternative services were necessary.[24] Nevertheless, it was important that such support services be developed in a nonhierarchical and nonmedical manner. Issues of power were always connected with issues of care. The discursive spaces offered by MNN and other publications allowed persons to talk about challenges in reentering their communities. In these foundational publications, the language of the liberation movement prefaced later discussions of rights.

As noted in the previous chapter's discussion of deinstitutionalization, the early mad liberation movement was crafted in a historical context where mental health care was moving out of the asylums and into the community. At the same time there were significant advances in the gay and lesbian movement, women's movement, and Black Power movement.[25] Many of the rights based concerns of this early movement were set against the hospital system and its forms of social control. Centered in major metropolitan areas such as San Francisco and New York, the mad liberation movement sought a range of intersectional rights from housing to the avoidance of coercive psychiatry. The quest for self-determination and voice formed the center of the movement.

The question of authority and self-definition is crucial to c/s/x activism, and Morrison describes this, drawing from bell hooks, as "the process of finding voice, speaking truth against power, finding that 'speaking center,' [by] claiming authority to speak rather than be spoken for (or spoken about) without representation of your point of view."[26] She states that "c/s/x group members are not endeavoring to be normal" but rather they are attempting to contest the authority to grant the category of normalcy to some persons and not to others.[27] The capacity for self-definition is at stake here, for example, whether one consents to be the object of psychiatric knowledge or insists on defining oneself as a subject. What ties together the diversity of c/s/x positions is the need to speak back to psychiatry and question its power. Morrison describes how

> some individuals returned to their doctors or hospitals for periodic crisis intervention, and others stayed as far as possible from the psychiatric establishment. Some worked in the mental health system as advocates for other patients or clients, and others insisted on a stronger voice in treatment. Some agitated for alternative treatments and/or the eradication of psychiatry, and others called for changes in the current health system to accommodate an increased voice for patients, clients, or "consumers." Some were on heavy doses of psychotropic medications that helped them function from day to day, and others rejected even the idea of such intervention for their problems in living.[28]

In this important quote Morrison underscores the range of perspectives and practical approaches inherent in c/s/x discourse, noting that the terms which one uses also implies a range of practical responses to psychiatry.

Language that one chooses to describe oneself is an important aspect of the operation of discourse. "Patient: I am a schizophrenic; Consumer: I am a person with schizophrenia; Survivor: I am a person who hears voices."[29] We could add one further interpretation: Ex-patient: I am a person who no longer hears voices. Presenting this schematically, the *patient* has an identity equivalent to the illness, the *consumer* has the ability to use services and negotiate with the system, and the *survivor* has an experience that has been stigmatized. Finally, the *ex-patient* has begun to exit the patient role. What is at stake in these discourse categories is the extent to which a person accepts mental illness as an identity.

At the same time, these are not discrete and unitary categories, but overlap, and as such each position is subject to negotiation with others and appropriation by outside experts.

The common thread between each strand of experience is a critique at the level of knowledge—how does the psychiatrist know who is sane and whose voice dominates in these discussions? This critique pertains to both official discourse and the settings in which this discourse is used.

In the discussion of these conceptual movements, we begin with the survivor perspective which is a radical point of view most closely allied with mad liberation, and turn toward the consumer movement and the recovery movement, which share common themes and still diverge from mad liberation. So even though the traditional acronym c/s/x states consumer/survivor/ex-patient, for conceptual reasons I approach them as survivor, consumer, and ex-patient movements.

The Survivor Movement and the Language of Rights

Working to deconstruct psychiatry and disprove its claims, activists have carried the themes of mad liberation into the twenty-first century under the rubric of survivorship. In 2001 psychologist Ron Bassman discussed his "incarceration" and "treatment" for schizophrenia in the pages of *Psychology Today*, and described himself as a "psychiatric survivor." He indicated that shock treatments "blasted huge holes in [his] memory, parts of which have never returned."[30] The term "survivor" is rooted in mad liberation, and it implies that so-called treatment has been harmful to people because it has hurt them physically and taken their rights away. Survivorship revives the two themes of advocacy and mutual support from mad liberation.

Emotional catharsis can be important to survivorship narratives. To return to Chamberlin's example for a moment, she describes benefiting from voicing her anger at the psychiatric establishment among likeminded peers. Claiming the name "survivor" rather than the status "victim" indicates that people have been able to catalyze their suffering into action.[31] Some who experience mental illness attribute it to traumatic events in their childhood,[32] but here the striking thing is that some people need to recover from the traumas incurred in treatment as well as the experience of mental illness.[33] Critic Sally Satel describes survivorship pejoratively: "The term survivor is not being used like the term 'cancer survivor,' someone who has had cancer and survived it, but rather like Holocaust survivor, someone who has been unjustly imprisoned and even tortured."[34] Understanding survivorship offers a profound revision of the meaning of psychiatric categories, focusing on the practices of psychiatry as implying a misuse of power.

Morrison studied the trajectory of survivor narratives through interviews she undertook at *Alternatives*, a major conference in the advocacy movement. Morrison notes the heroic nature of survivorship stories. Some advocates entered the mental health system with a mixture of trust and mistrust (only a few were involuntarily committed), and many told stories of having their personal life goals discredited by the psychiatric system, such as being told that they could not accomplish their educational objectives.[35] In the face of such disparagement, many engaged in resistance, and experienced solidarity by sharing their narratives. In these narratives, she notes that many survivors challenge their doctors over the expectations of chronicity and relate experiences of dehumanization and diminishment by psychiatrists. These experiences range from differences of opinion to the invalidation that can often be communicated in nonverbal terms, as noted in the Rosenhan study in the previous chapter. Some examples include being mocked, having one's goals derided, and being diminished in a variety of ways. Less explicit marginalization can take place as psychiatrists silence patient's descriptions of their delusions and the psychiatric framework is underscored.[36]

They manifested ambivalence about the medical system, some continuing to use medication to "take the edge off" and others negotiating with their doctors to have doses lowered for particular purposes.[37] Some patients accepted psychotropic medications but resisted medication and other forms of treatment such as ECT. One mental health user argued for a lower dosage of psychotropic medications with his doctor by stating, "Please, because I am active across the state in advocacy, I have to keep my head cleared up."[38] Others described "work[ing] through [problems] prayerfully and with some close friends and family" before they talked to a psychiatrist.[39] In some cases, educated advocates earned their release from mental hospitals by arguing with judges about their condition.

Morrison notes that many of the survivor narratives she heard involved a "coming to consciousness" about what one had experienced by being in a community of like-minded others who were able to talk about their oppression. Note the importance of partner-participants who are able to hear these narratives. Part of what counts for survivors is expressing anger and outrage about elements of their psychiatric treatment rather than focusing the blame inward by taking on themes of a perceived flaw, unworthiness, or having been damaged.

Survivorship often connotes endurance, thus indicating that what has been survived can be a significant trauma—being given shock treatments as a six-year-old, as in the story of Ted Chabasinki, a man who has gone on to advocate for children in the psychiatric system[40]—or it can be the dehumanization of being spoken about as if one does not exist, being interrupted or ignored, and being dismissed despite the fact that one has a valuable and worthwhile perspective to share. Survivor narratives bear a close resemblance to advocacy since they seem to catalyze the anger of collective identity into change that can be used to the benefit of others. At the center of the survivor category is a profound critique of the psychiatric system and its knowledge.

Survivorship has moved from a silenced reality to a public identity through the language of rights. In recent years elements of a critical survivor movement has had an influence on public knowledge and intervention about mental illness at a global level. This survivor movement has linked the language of rights with the language of self-definition and self-determination. As Morrison notes, leading figures from mad liberation groups such as MindFreedom International—have achieved consulting NGO status to the United Nations and members have been nominated to the UN Ad Hoc committee on disability and human rights.[41] Building on a tradition that Chamberlin established when she linked rights to the preservation of viable alternatives, the rights language was important when a person's dignity had been systematically denied and when people had been confused with their illness, thereby stripping away their rights or treating them like children. Addressing stigma is one possible approach to increasing compassion for persons who have been through the psychiatric system. Another is shifting the categories of knowledge away from implicit sanism and mentalism toward more inclusive models.

According to one c/s/x advocate, having rights means, "[being] regarded as a full human being... able to define one's own identity and celebrate this identity in various ways."[42] Significant movements have emerged that have begun to link rights across various forms of oppression, from the disability that comes from social exclusion (a social disability approach) to the oppression of racism and sexism and heterosexism. In order for people to define their public identities they often need the leisure that comes from having appropriate work, voice, and right to democratic process. Efforts in Sweden to give psychiatric patients a right to vote, for example, indicate that citizenship is often at stake in mental health rights based organizing.[43] At the same time, there are challenges faced in the nexus between disability organizing and mental health advocacy. Understanding the intersections between various forms of oppression requires conceptualizing the difference between impairment and disability.

Many people who have been diagnosed with mental illness face disability of some kind, but they often resist the label of disabled, perhaps because of a limited understanding of that term. Social disability means a lack of access to the social sphere rather than a functional impairment. John Swinton explains this distinction: "impairments are 'the discrete functional limitations that are present within individuals that cause some manifestations of physical, mental or sensory impedance. Disability relates to the loss or limitation of opportunities to take part in the normal life of the community on an equal level with others due to physical and/or social barriers.'"[44] According to a social disability model, disability is constructed and "people are disabled by society's reaction to impairment," and for this reason disability is a social reality rather than an absence of some kind of capacity.[45] Some c/s/x activists have challenged the connection to disability, eschewing the language of intellectual disability.[46] This is a sign of the movement's own ableism and an indication that the rights perspective has not been completely integrated. Disability does not imply impairment, but is a social construct having to do with access and self-determination.

The intersection between disability and mental illness is complex. In an essay written by psychiatric survivors Peter Beresford, Gloria Gifford, and Chris Harrison, the authors note that "disability and distress seem to be perceived differently... Disability in a union meeting gets access, but so far there is not the same recognition of survivors' rights and needs around mental distress."[47] Given that economic oppression often causes mental disability, this lack of awareness has profound consequences. Some psychiatric survivors, such as Bassman, claim that they have been disabled by being treated with shock treatments for their mental distress, so that their disability does not come from a supposed organically caused mental illness but rather how they have been treated for it.

The language of rights and themes from disability studies have been reclaimed recently by c/s/x activists with a strong orientation around survivorship. A group of Mindfreedom activists gathered in 2000 and 2001 in Highlander, Tennessee to draft a call to action based upon the language of rights that links up with social critiques of disability. In this statement, they insisted that being a survivor was akin to other forms of intersectionality such being a minority, a disabled person, gay, lesbian, or transgendered person, or "people forced to live in poverty among the great wealth and abundance of the corporate economy." They lived realities that resulted in social oppression that did not stem from inherent characteristics but lack of access and opportunities.[48] Note the importance of income inequality in the advocacy work of this social group devoted to the rights of those who have encountered the mental health system. While new legislation sought to make it easier to coerce someone to take medication outside the hospital, this group "fight[s] against the passage and implementation of legislation making it easier to lock up, shock, and forcibly drug people labeled with psychiatric disorders" and to build, by contrast, a system that fosters "self-determination."[49] The path to these rights, for the MindFreedom group, was that people would "heal each other by telling [their] stories."[50] This statement emphasizes a strong sense of community and collective responsibility for shared narratives.

The term "psychiatric survivor" emphasizes the conditions of psychiatric confinement and hospitalization in order to develop a collective identity that resists the patient category by narrative means. Just as activists who resisted the widespread use of ECT described their campaign as a struggle for memory, the survivor identity engages in resistance, negotiation, and sometimes outright rejection of the treatments of psychiatry in order to craft a space of subjectivity beyond the subject–object dichotomy of psychiatric power.[51]

Activism in this field is different from simply claiming an alternative identity as a point of pride. C/s/x activists also wrest the power of self-definition away from psychiatry by challenging the disease model of mental illness. Under the subject–object dichotomy of psychiatry, the mental health expert is the subject who has knowledge over the patient's life, the text of which becomes an object to the psychiatrist by reading symptoms. The contrary space offered by the term *survivor* runs the risk of reifying the identity of a person who has been psychiatrized by emphasizing the nature of psychiatric trauma in an ongoing fashion, but it is not at the risk of forgetting. It is difficult to claim pride over a label someone has given you, so pride is frequently taken in renaming or recasting that label.

Survivors frequently challenge the theme of chronicity. If people who have been diagnosed as severely mentally ill and hospitalized for it feel shame and hide this experience, it is often because they believe that recovery is impossible. Yet Bassman deconstructs this logic: "Such reasoning makes me and my peers look like exceptions" since they include functioning professionals and working-class people who did not wear their psychiatric histories on their sleeves.[52] Bassman argued that they were not exceptions at all, but that the treatment they received from psychiatry, along with the shame that persists in discussing mental health treatment, led to a two-fold silencing of the experience. Survivorship is one possible way of breaking that silence.

Chamberlin indicated that naming oneself with a psychiatric survivor status could be a doorway to expanding the narratives of one's life. Just as Bassman suggested that people kept their experience of mental hospitalization quiet because of perceived shame, Chamberlin argues that discussing hospitalization more openly can challenge the secrecy and alleviate the shame surrounding this phenomenon. It can also lead to people building coalitions that help address problematic aspects of the mental health system. This can be done simply by naming the range of experiences of mental distress and suffering and discussing psychiatric histories, and it can alternatively offer solidarity across these shared narratives.

This kind of movement addresses a common experience of psychiatric survivors: many cease to trust their own judgments and feel a kind of shame when they leave the hospital. This is partly because of internalized mentalism, reinforced by the notion of chronicity. The problem with chronicity for some survivors is that it leads to a foreshortening of stories, a kind of narrative truncation, in which the person loses the capacity to interpret and determine their own experience and instead becomes subject to the experience/interpretation of the other.[53] The stories of resistance, negotiation, and meaning-making fall into the background while the symptom or syndrome is what is treated in the foreground. When we begin to understand these various positions, we can see how they show up in the language of self-definition, those terms that people use to describe themselves and their experience.

Consumer Movement

The consumer category came to being in the 1980s in the United States. A Republican government came into power that could be described as "neoliberal." Republicans accepted self-help groups but simultaneously reduced financial support for social services in general. Using the language of mad liberation to further defund mental health care, the government accepted peer-support terminology while refusing to fiscally support the state run community mental health centers that were supposed to provide mental health care across regions of the United States.[54] This insidious shift left fewer community supports in place for homeless people or the transinstitutionalized.

In the gap left by neoliberalism's gutting of mental health care, there was the new rhetoric of the consumer. Within this political climate, mental health care was shifted by the powerful language of groups such as NAMI that educated the community about mental illness as a brain disease and the person with mental illness as a user of mental health services. A person who took medication inhabited a complex kind of identity—now a user who could be invited onto boards of mental health organizations—but also a consumer who was responsible to manage their health. Often users borrowed "persons with" language from disability advocacy so that the individuals were seen as more than the disease.[55]

This shift led to a split between activists who felt that the new emphasis on user involvement was co-optation and those who wanted a voice at the table in treatment decisions. Chamberlin puts it thus, "I've never been sure where the term 'consumer' came from...this new label...was certainly more comfortable for professionals than 'mental patient,' 'survivor,' or 'inmate,' (which were meant, in part, to be disquieting)."[56]

In the managed care era choice was a key aspect of health care so that being a consumer meant having a marketplace from which to choose one's health care options. Being a consumer meant, on the one hand, being someone who takes drugs and other treatments and also someone who has an influence over the quality of services. The status of "consumer" or "user" of mental health services often included an element of consciousness-raising, since persons who participate in user movements tend to understand their rights as mental patients and have studied how to intervene in situations in which their rights are being denied.[57] Although this emphasis on choice was implied in the title consumer, the actual stress was laid upon cost effectiveness and efficiency in managed care rather than what occurred for the good of the patient.

Paradoxically, the term consumer seems to presume a capacity for equal participation that may only have come as the result of gains made by the earlier liberation movement. An important shift took place between mad liberation discourse and consumer rhetoric. The term consumer movement implies that participants are at equal levels and have the same resources to participate in a public conversation about mental health care, whereas, because of the intersectional nature of oppression, this is seldom true. The presumption of an equality that is not actually present is a key theme of the neoliberal era. Persons with more money, who are white, and who are male, have *de facto* more power in society and by extension more control over their mental health treatment. Unfortunately, minority clients are most likely to receive high doses of medication and much less likely to receive psychotherapy "than white service users."[58] It seems that the more social power one has in a given situation, the more capable one is of becoming a consumer of one's health care.

At the same time, there is another perspective from which to critique the notion of consumer. Without a real range of health care options (alternatives, psychotherapy, and medication), and without the capacity to access these options, the idea of choice is a mirage. Nevertheless, note how the stress in this movement came to be laid upon consumption as choice at the very moment in which, as the previous two chapters suggested, the working rights of average Americans and their pay was declining and in which people were being defined vis-à-vis a biomedical model of mental illness. Under managed care, options were systematically curtailed just as persons were positioned as consumers (rather than critics or workers, for example).

The rise of the consumer era presaged a shift in mad liberation organizing. In 1986 Madness Network News closed, with its final publication including two simultaneously published endings:

> First ending: Very few anti-psychiatry projects remain. But one thing is certain, no matter how unorganized the movement may currently appear in the public... resistance to psychiatric assault and psychiatric oppression will continue to grow. Psychiatry will one day be abolished.[59]

On the other hand, a second skeptical ending was published,

> Second ending: A lack of real communication and trust in recent years among people has been another major cause for this success [in co-opting the movement] and continues to jeopardize what is left of our movement... Very few anti-psychiatry projects remain. Those that do tend to be isolated. It remains to be seen whether or not a visible, organized anti-psychiatry movement will continue to exist at this time.[60]

The capacity to hold these two endings in tension, refusing to redact either one, indicates the tension in the c/s/x movement at this point. As the identity politics movements of the 1960s and 1970s began to lose voice, the marketplace became the most salient reality, leading to a shift away from survivorship toward consumer identities.

The consumer movement's emphasis was on reform rather than abolition and a "seat at the table" rather than overturning the table.[61] In boardrooms and legislative hearings, the voices of users were making an impact.[62] While the movement shifted to policy change and development, many organizations were renamed and given federal dollars. Beneficiaries included the earlier liberation activists such as Joseph Rogers, whose Mental Health Consumers' Self-Help Clearinghouse became a beneficiary of these federal dollars. Some consumer groups offered oversight to particular state hospitals and brought in outside observers to audit them. The Conference on Human Rights and Psychiatric Oppression became Alternatives, which was now funded by federal monies.

The consumer movement in the 1980s was accompanied by another movement that has sometimes paired with it—the National Alliance for the Mentally Ill (NAMI), a group that claimed to speak for persons with mental illness even as it advocated for coercive hospitalization laws. NAMI's advocacy has included empowering families to fight for budget dollars for mental health services and yet it has coincided with other epistemological shifts that were perceived by some in the mad liberation movement as crises of representation. On the one hand, NAMI offered a "stigma-busting" approach to mental illness that "coincided with strengthened 'brain disorder' models of mental illness."[63] The stigma busting helpfully critiques much pejorative language about people diagnosed with mental illness and the overestimation of their dangerousness. Such advocacy is helpful.

Yet at the same time, NAMI promoted "campaigns for more forced treatment" and claimed to be the "nation's voice on mental illness" even as it was guided primarily by the voices of family members rather than survivors. Even the kind of knowledge upon which its resources were based emphasized biomedical factors that reduced mental illness to a brain disease rather than the result of oppression or a source of knowledge. In the attempt to foster a non-stigma inducing approach to mental illness, the NAMI organization simultaneously sponsored a one-dimensional picture of it. This approach supposedly relies upon reducing the shame or stigma of mental illness by equating it with physical illness, yet this system also reproduced some of the factual inaccuracies of the "chemical imbalance" theory at a public level. Pharmaceutical corporations, whose rise was described in the previous chapter, have funded this group heavily. Mad liberation's social explanations of mental illness are pushed aside by a pharmaceutically sponsored approach to brain disease.

Consumerism in mental health care seems to rely upon models of equal access and choice for a presumably neoliberal subject, but this approach has tended to silence voices of mad liberation. Why is this the case? The consumer framework itself presumed that the epistemological status of psychiatry was sound and argued for access to treatment based on this model. The important gains in this area were made in the greater inclusion of mental health users into the oversight of mental health institutions, where users were invited to be on corporate boards and public policy decisions. The risk was that these voices were co-opted by others. Chamberlin indicated that the public groups tended to prefer "good" consumers who did not critique psychiatric ideas. Theorists in the United Kingdom have likewise brought a critical perspective to the consumer term, since the ability to be a consumer often seemed like a mirage. "Consumerist rhetoric is often cynically mobilized to undermine workers (and arguably survivor's) collective interests."[64] Those who would "consume" or "use" mental health services had their service options "restricted by geographical location, ability to pay, class, gender, race, ethnicity, and age." The authors acknowledge that the term consumer refers to some kind of "quest for self-determination," but argue that its ambiguity is dangerous.[65]

Under neoliberalism the market has infiltrated all aspects of society and no one has benefited more from this rise than from pharmaceutical corporations who have been among the most successful neoliberal entrepreneurs. As a part of this change, during the 1990s the decade of the brain reinserted a biomedical model of mental illness in full force, along with guidelines for making sure that all people had access to mental treatment in the community, which included a Program for Assertive Community Treatment (PACT), in which people would be forced to take medication in their homes. The notion of being a mental health user or consumer, with the positive elements of choice and decision making, shaded easily into outpatient programs that resulted in forced medication. Under managed care in the 1990s, "consumer satisfaction teams" were instituted to obtain feedback about services and change delivery systems; this positive change was balanced by a turn toward the biomedicalization of mental illness. Most nationally funded research was now devoted to discovering the organic basis of mental illness. Including the consumer perspectives had become fashionable, yet a fundamental critique of the conceptual status of mental illness, along with a criticism of the practices, discourse, and social location of psychiatry, seemed ever more remote. Well-established research facts, such as the contribution of poverty to a range of mental distress, have been downplayed in research emphasizing organic causes and brain imbalance. Consumer groups have sponsored this research.

At the same time, the consumer rights movement did allow for greater voice and participation at the level of state government, public policy, and in the quality control of mental health institutions. This gain seems to have been bought at the price of softening the critique of the more radical wing of the movement, namely, the critique that mental illness was either social control or meaningful adaptation to an unworkable social situation. In this section I have argued that the consumer movement presupposes a framework of access based on a neoliberal version of the self: its important gains were increasing representation on committees and boards for mental health. Even if this was simply a shift in language, it was important. Nevertheless, this greater representation did not necessarily lead to greater capacity for self-definition or self-determination.

Ex-Patients, Structural Factors, and the Need for Narration

Several meta-analyses of patients with schizophrenia over 20 years in the United States found that one-half to two-thirds of these persons had "achieved recovery or significant improvement," and this was a substantially agreed-upon conclusion drawn across the literature.[66] The possibility of recovery is an emerging notion in the field of mental health that has begun to be pursued in popular texts. Nevertheless, in institutions where a biomedical model dominates, with organic and brain explanations at the fore and pharmacological solutions considered the only conceivable treatment, the notion that people could significantly recover from mental illness has been a negligible part of the conversation.

In interviews with Swedish ex-patients, Alain Topor analyzed factors that lead to recovery from mental illness: economic stability; positive relationships with helping professionals who shared some of their real, human selves with clients; and meaningful peer relationships.[67] The term ex-patient implies that one has exited significantly from the role of the mental patient. Exploring a term coined by survivors, Topor discusses what it takes to exit the role of a mental patient, using Fuchs Ebaugh's discussion of role-exit.

In order for a person to envision exiting a role (such as the role of a patient) there has to be a perceptible ending to a state, a sense of voluntariness, and the prospect of reversibility. Discovering that the "centrality of the role" in the person's life contributed significantly to their capacity for exiting that role. Often an important role has to be replaced with other roles. This is important for ministers and other counselors who may seek to help persons discover elements of their identity beyond the disease category.

Topor states that no one expects mental illness recovery, and that this pessimism contributes to difficulties for individuals who have been diagnosed with mental illness. He notes this social pessimism—"The most people in this situation can expect is to become an 'ex,' a term that implies the continuing existence of a latent problem; they remain an 'ex' *with no possibility to become anything else.*"[68] As such, even the notion of becoming an ex-patient is fraught with possible contradictions, in part because it is such an unusual idea to persons who have accepted a biomedical framework alone.

Topor discovered that family also had to go through a process of role-exit when their family members recovered from what was presumed to be a chronic condition. As the result of longitudinal study of many nations, the World Health Organization (WHO) discovered that nations with the greatest income equality saw the highest rates of recovery from mental illness. Around 10 to 20 percent of people diagnosed with schizophrenia recovered completely from and around 30 to 40 percent experienced a significant diminishment of their symptoms so they were able to function. Rates of recovery were negatively correlated with the rate of unemployment in the entire society.[69] One of the things that seemed to lead to a successful recovery from mental illness was the notion that schizophrenia had only impacted some parts of a person's personality and that other parts of their personality had remained largely intact.[70]

A key aspect of exiting the role of a mental patient is a form of narrative revision, undertaken in community, in which one gains greater conceptual control over the factors that influence one's life. Arguments could be made that these revisions begin with the central experience of mental illness diagnosis. Given Kleinman's reflections on losing a social world through diagnosis in the previous chapter, we can see this as the starting point for new kinds of storytelling. Just at the point a patient loses a world through diagnosis, they must develop their own through narration.

Another researcher in the United Kingdom found that "many considered themselves ill only when they were unable to cope with their problems" and that nobody used medication as their only coping strategy. Indeed, when asked, people preferred to discuss their own coping strategies first and also noted how they used their coping strategies even in relationship with medication management.[71] This could be done by splitting apart the inner world and arrogating illness to one part while preserving another part from harm—some form of this is frequently done in psychiatry already by seeing some part of the patient as containing "delusions" that should not be colluded with.⁷² However, another option is to critique such splitting altogether.

Ex-patients also noted that an important part of the recovery process was a relationship with a helping person. This could be someone with whom they could negotiate medication and its side effects, echoing the research in the previous chapter about the importance of nonspecific factors such as the patient–physician relationship in the recovery from mental illness. The most helpful partner was not a professional, but a peer who had been through a similar experience.

Widespread social poverty directly impacted the quantity and length of hospital admissions. As we saw in Warner's exploration of the WHO statistic, there was a strong correlation between unemployment and the rates of recovery from schizophrenia.⁷³ Understanding this seldom-acknowledged statistic means that even as there is a biological basis for schizophrenia, social factors play a significant role in its onset and course. Mental illnesses involve social class—recall Chamberlin's insistence that upper-class psychiatrists may have little acquaintance with the daily stresses experienced by poor patients—and poverty has a direct role to play in mental illness treatment. According to Topor, elements such as economic inequity and social class have a direct bearing on psychological recovery. It is therefore necessary to see the social world and the experience of mental illness as overlapping significantly, so that to leave a macro-analysis out of the experience of mental illness results in an "extremely unbalanced" conception of disease.⁷⁴

Hearing Voices

Once people are able to exit the patient role to some extent they often wish to talk with others about the experience of active coping and making sense of their lives. Challenging the traditional understanding of pathology as presented in the taxonomies of the DSM, persons seeking to exit the patient role make positive meaning of experiences that the DSM labels as "symptomatic." While hearing voices has been considered a symptom of mental illness, the MIND group in the United Kingdom has argued that it is actually a meaningful experience to people and much more widespread than previously thought.⁷⁵ Hearing voices, or "clairaudience" has typically been described as one of the "positive" aspects of schizophrenia, as compared with "negative" elements such as withdrawal. Understanding the importance of hearing voices as a broad ranging phenomenon toward which different meanings can be placed, it becomes apparent that there are multiple ways to narrate experiences that have been deemed as symptoms by traditional psychiatry.

In the United Kingdom the *Hearing Voices* movement, pioneered by the group MIND, has begun to study this experience beyond the psychiatric label. These "extrasensory perceptions" were heard by many in the population who did not identify as patients, had never been hospitalized, and never would be. MIND, a group that began 60 years ago in the United Kingdom, rejects pharmaceutical sponsorship and foregrounds user narratives, and they have published several volumes that explore these phenomenon.[76]

At issue was meaning making—how might persons who heard voices make sense of their experiences? As such, once the deconstructive work of mad liberation had begun, there emerged a need to interpret a range of experiences that were otherwise silenced. This might be described as a further step in identity consolidation. Making meaning fills a major space in the process of becoming an ex-patient because it returns naming-rights to persons who have gone through their experiences of mental distress. In the United Kingdom several recent anthologies describe hearing voices in c/s/x terms, and the work in the analysis that follows will be drawn from their accounts.

Some authors described hearing voices as having an element of spirituality. Since ministers and counselors frequently discuss religious matters with people, it is fitting to acknowledge this aspect of c/s/x discourse. This is especially important because many c/s/x advocates, especially those who are racial minorities, describe spirituality as being important to them.[77] Some understood the voices as representing guiding spirits, citing the process of discerning these spirits as even including classical aspects of the spiritual journey: illumination, purgation, and union.[78] Noting how talking about religion violates the principles of a presumably secular society, one activist in the United Kingdom stated, "It was a bit of cheek to arrest me for talking about God."[79]

Mental health users who had premonitions of the physical illnesses of others had to learn to manage these intuitions. One psychiatric survivor, given the pseudonym Rachel, described nightmares of going to her own funeral and terrible images in her head telling her "you need help."[80] After being hospitalized for psychiatric illness, she found out that she did have cancer and felt that this is what her voices were trying to communicate in the first place.[81] Others described how they needed to learn to cope even with the positive aspects of voices: "I came to realize that I should not rely on voices to help me in matters I was quite capable of sorting out myself."[82] Children with active imaginations, who had childhood fantasy friends that spoke with them, finally realized that they should no longer talk about these childhood friends and their voices. Note that persons tended to experience some congruence between their voices and their world: it is not as though voices were completely alien to their experience. In Zanzibar, for example, a young woman from a Muslim family heard voices urging her to be modest.[83]

The content of voices can be related to the cultural trauma of a particular era. For example, a woman who lived through both world wars described hearing voices about the war. Likewise, at the beginning of the Gulf War a man heard voices that were calling for blood, perhaps reflecting the collective trauma of a culture at war in an individual's mind.[84] One young woman whose parents were of different ethnicities and who had faced bullying and racist teasing described how her own struggle to be known showed up in her mental difficulties. In terms that echo Fanon's powerful critique in the previous chapter, she concluded "Any mental health professional will only help me if he or she understands racism" since "my mental health, race, and culture are intrinsically linked."[85] This is not to suggest that there was some quality related to her race that led her to be mentally ill, but rather the oppression of a racist society contributed to traumatic stress. One person described how the voices they heard encouraged them to get involved in Civil Rights activism. Another told of being forced into hospitalization after protesting against the conservative party of the UK government. As such, no dividing line exists among culture, power, and clairaudience. This phenomenon often relates directly to the wider culture and interacts with power.

At the same time, people frequently understood their experiences of clairaudience as including negative aspects and requiring active coping skills. This led the group to ask the question of coping, "How it might be possible to manage the hearing of voices without becoming a psychiatric patient?"[86] Answering such questions could lead users to develop coping skills that helped them. An initial step was recognizing a voice as negative. One c/s/x activist described a voice as negative if it "stopped me from doing things or did things to me."[87] Recognizing a voice as negative often involved a discernment that was psychological in nature. Using psychological language, one survivor described how the negative voices "could be a projection from one's own unconscious" that "play[ed] upon fears" and they described how they learned, drawing tools from parapsychology, guided meditation, and visualization, to define and limit the role that the negative voices would play in their lives.[88] One author noted that it was important to have a strong identity in order to work well with the negative voices, emphasizing the importance of psychological factors such as work. Some insights included the confrontation with negative voices, setting them aside, or "rejecting" elements that were unhelpful. Authors described needing to respond to negative voices with some kind of "counterforce" that would limit their range and influence.

Authors actively engaged voices at times in order to manage their intensity. This included setting aside some limited time of day to listen to these voices and then progressively shrinking the time given to them. One author linked the experience of negative voices to stress and suggested that she could completely stop the voices if she decided not to take any further risks at work, but that this approach was unacceptable as an alternative because work mattered too much. Persons in the Hearing Voices movement have attempted to popularize their knowledge in accessible books and websites and they have encouraged ex-patients to talk about their experience together in order to share knowledge.[89] The Hearing Voices movement is one manifestation of the self-representation of c/s/x advocates who take the description of their mental distress into their own hands. This movement that has been furthered by the advent of the Internet and the capacity to self-publish.

One author, Richie B., publishing in the United Kingdom, *Speaking Our Minds* series described how important it was to discover his sexual abuse by his alcoholic father and the central role that trauma played in his life. For him, the trauma category came to *replace* the category of schizophrenia: it was not that schizophrenia was simply a "risk" that came from trauma, but that trauma came to take the place of mental illness as the story of what happened to him, bringing the suffering of trauma to the forefront and placing the consequent suffering of schizophrenia in the background.[90] Biomedical mental illness models have often been critiqued for missing "life events" or "spiritual crises" altogether, hence it is the role of the c/s/x advocates to make sure these stories are told and heard.[91]

Another author links his mental suffering directly with the social system, discussing "the miracle the world has been praying for... the drug to cure the world of capitalism."[92] He describes his own experience as an "inferno kindled by the rubbing together of grinding poverty and wealth."[93] This author talked about the psychiatric pressure to accept a biomedical model for illness, stating, "They want me to stop searching."[94] The same author used religious themes of identification, stating that the author felt protected by God and also felt Christ's identification with him, stating, "You bear his stripes for what you are."[95] The context in which suffering is experienced is simultaneously macroeconomic, personal, and religious, indicating that the experience of mental suffering is a complex and multidimensional reality in which one category is not all explanatory.

Ex-patients use stories to interpret their illnesses, and in the exploration of both the Hearing Voices movement, there have been a range of narratives that have involved spiritual themes, collective trauma, discussions of race, war, and activism, and even critiques of capitalism. Fundamentally, what emerges in these discussions is the sense of voices-in-context rather than disembodied symptoms or universal categories. This leads to the fundamental tension between psychiatric perspectives and of c/s/x activists.

C/s/x activists' stories are broadly varied and rooted in a variety of forms of practical action so it is difficult to summarize them in an oversimplified fashion. One way of exploring the tensions is to look at what biomedical psychiatry—focused solely on the brain and genes for organic causes of mental suffering and their amelioration—inadequately addresses. For one thing, it denies the complete context of a person's life: trauma-based symptoms are typically ignored. Social exclusion and denial of employment opportunities are underemphasized. Poverty is almost entirely neglected. Another crucial point is that a consumer category that places the mental illness identity in the foreground rather than other intersectional identities—such as one's identity as a woman, as a minority, or as a working-class person—risks a kind of reductionism. If mental illness is the primary theme, then the social suffering of the economic world and social world elide to the background.

Philosophically, biomedical psychiatry follows the lead of Karl Jaspers, who, in his *General Psychopathology* supposed you could separate off questions of value and have a simple science of the mind. This "methodological individualism" of psychiatry leads to the notion that you could study a patient to discover the answer to the question "What is mental illness?"[96] In this form of Cartesianism, body and mind have been dualistically posited against each other, with an individual mind speaking directly to an incontrovertible truth about a person. This Cartesian tradition has continued with the new emphasis of listening to the language of people diagnosed with schizophrenia for "poverty of speech" or various levels of "expressed emotion" that fall outside the range of presumed normality.[97] Scholars have analyzed the racial normativity in discussions of expressed emotion, and the presumed poverty of speech of schizophrenics belies a broader material poverty, shared by many, in a neoliberal capitalist economy.[98]

In much literature on mental illness, professional viewpoints dominate. A range of psychological interventions imply this epistemological standpoint. For example, as cognitivists look for the internal schema from which the talk of psychotics arises, or as researchers on "expressed emotion" study the speech of schizophrenics for ruptures in it, they are exploring behaviors and symptoms at an individual level that can supposedly be read in light of the psychological theory. Psychiatric theories frequently stigmatize difference rather than appreciating it and learning from it.

Methodological individualism does not completely countenance the rich complexity of narratives such as those heard in the Hearing Voices movement. When the power of knowledge lies entirely with a medical model, there is little room for a discussion of the power of such marginalized knowledge, for example, the ongoing impact of racism on mental health care. The consequences of this is an implicit blaming of the survivor—one who has already suffered from multiple oppressions now has the new oppression of a psychiatric identity placed upon them. Psychiatric symptoms are much more richly connected to culture, spirituality, social class, and social location.

People engaged in c/s/x advocacy reclaim their voices from biomedical psychiatry, sharing important narratives that center on peer support, self-definition, and self-determination. In focusing on peer support, advocates highlight that persons who have faced mental distress are uniquely positioned to support one another. Through an emphasis on self-definition, advocates argue that people have a right to tell their own story and make sense of it within a logic that coheres for their own mind. By stressing self-determination, advocates declare that people need a chance to live according to the meanings that they would choose for their lives, which also includes full access to important goods such as food, shelter, education, and opportunity.

A quantitative study from the United Kingdom run by c/s/x advocates found that peer support was the most helpful aspect of mental health care, trumping both medication and psychotherapy. Among the most pressing needs was simply *someone you could talk with*, who would show compassion toward what you say in the context in which your conversation occurred. This support was often found among peers who had been through a similar experience and who expressed acceptance and understanding. Additionally, those who had experienced homelessness or financial distress listed money as an important need. Likewise, spiritual needs were significant to many users, which led the researchers to conclude,

> The feeling of being loved by God unconditionally—"warts and all"—was an important aspect of God's presence for some people. They believed God would continue to be there for them no matter what happened in their lives and regardless of their illness or distress. A feeling of being loved unconditionally by God was particularly important to people who were socially isolated or lonely.[99]

As we can see, themes of religiosity and spirituality are closely connected to mental illness identity, so that through naming one's experience of stigma and oppressive struggle one has an opportunity to more closely experience God. This friendship and intimacy can be strengthened if outsiders learn some of the conceptual categories behind c/s/x activism and the needs of this community. The quote noted previously indicates that one of the primary needs is a relationship that conveys God's unconditional love.

Coercive Psychiatry

As we have seen, the capacity for self-definition is one part of advocacy. Another part is the fostering of conditions in which people would be able to exercise their self-definition. One of the important issues in the c/s/x movement is the issue of autonomy and access, which may be viewed as a continuum. On the side of autonomy, persons in the movement argue that their rights are violated when they are forced to undergo treatment that they do not choose. On the side of access, some advocate for the ability to utilize mental health care in communities where there are few supports for those suffering from mental distress.

Legal discussions of responsibility and mental health have shifted over the years. Landmark decisions such as O'Connor versus Donaldson (1975) and Rogers versus Okin (1982) ruled that coercive treatment was unlawful unless people were determined to be a threat to themselves and others.[100] In a series of studies, Dershowitz found that psychiatrists overestimated the dangerousness of people suffering from mental distress.[101] The controversy has expanded with the Programs for Aggressive Community Treatment (PACT), a program that is implemented in several states, that forces people who live in halfway houses or their own home to take medication or be placed in mental hospitals again. Mind Freedom and other groups have fought forced treatment by challenging the stereotypes of those suffering from mental distress. The courts continue to be venues where self-determination struggles are fought between persons diagnosed with mental illness and the wider society.

At issue in the entire debate is the question of whether coercion is ever justifiable in care. Swedish ethicist Tännsjö defines coercion in medicine as occurring "When, intentionally, through the use of force, or threats, or manipulation, or positive incentives (or gratifications), the person is made to accept (or simply to undergo) a certain treatment he or she does not want to undergo (in the absence of the force, the threat, or the incentives, or gratifications)."[102] He argues that conceptual uncertainty about the effectiveness of psychiatric medicine, their limited effectiveness in some cases, and the autonomy of persons diagnosed with mental illness as subjects makes such coercion untenable from an ethical point of view.

One lens to examine this debate more closely is the lens of disability studies. Scholar Tina Minkowitz argued that the landmark *Convention on the Rights of Persons with Disabilities* established that it is unjust to take away the liberty of persons with disabilities. She classed psychiatrized people as disabled and argued that society should stop the process of coercion and instead respond with a truth and reconciliation commission that unveils the oppression committed by psychiatry. If we link the experience of radical or social disability—not functional impedance but rather a lack of social access, often deepened by aspects of psychiatric treatment itself—then it makes sense to safeguard the autonomy of people who have been diagnosed with mental illness.

Assessing the liberties of psychiatric people should be done in ways that balance needs and social goods. To return again briefly to Tännsjö's argument, he maintains that the need of the patient that justifies psychiatric intervention is only in the case of a life being harmed. In many instances persons who are deemed unable to "make an autonomous decision" are coercively treated against their will.[103] Citing the *Convention on Human Rights and Biomedicine* in the European Union, he argues for what he terms the "Life Rescue" model and maintains that only the drugs that are seen as preserving a person's life should be given coercively. If a person refuses medication to treat their mental illness, then their rights should be honored, following the 1982 decision in the United States in Rogers versus Commissioner of Department of Mental Health described earlier.[104]

Tännsjö rejects the argument that persons diagnosed with mental illness need to be protected from their own decisions since we do not know their best interests. He also indicates that the medication for mental illness has been questioned both on the grounds of efficacy and on the grounds that they change the personality of the person suffering. In his estimation, the possibility that either of these arguments hold up is enough to preclude forced psychotropic medication for persons with mental distress.

He argues persuasively that people should have their lives preserved. Yet if they rejected medication they should not have medication forced upon them. They should have had a veto just like they do in somatic medicine. If stigma contributes to the view of mentally ill persons as dangerous, and this vision of dangerousness makes it so that persons' rights are violated, then this is unethical.

Against the backdrop of the discussion of deinstitutionalization in the previous chapter, such theorizing may only make sense in social contexts where there is already a great deal of support for individuals in communities, such as Tännsjö's home country of Sweden. In the United States, where people are largely left to fend for themselves and in which society is not tolerant of different behaviors, a period of emotional suffering may lead to one becoming homeless or being hospitalized, or being put into prison. In this case, mental illness involves social position, such as social class, gender, and race.

There is another difficulty with Tännsjö's argument. Issues of coercion and care are rarely divisible into discrete physical and mental realms. As I have noted already it is important to reject the false Cartesianism of psychiatry. The body and mind are inextricably linked. When a person no longer brushes their teeth or bathes as a result of not taking psychiatric medications, they sometimes enter the health care system in which their physical needs such as infections are met by hospitals. On the other hand, their psychiatric medications may give them what they consider unacceptable side effects. Linking the notion of mind and body in c/s/x activism means that physical needs and mental needs may have to be balanced in the discussion of the ultimate goods toward which a person may be persuaded. Someone off their medications may be able to speak, reason, and advocate more clearly, but may lack the proper self-care and hygiene to keep them healthy in a bodily sense so that they are judged to be harming themselves. In these cases the Life Rescue model may necessitate intervention even if they are not a danger to themselves based on their thoughts.

Tännsjö's principles apply here again. He argues that principles for the autonomy of the individual should be met in all possible circumstances and that cases when it is not should be "*kept at a minimum.*"[105]

When it is not possible, it should be for the person's own benefit that circumstances are changed, not for the benefit of others. The first option should always be persuasion rather than coercion, yet he notes that he realizes how often the principles of the Convention are violated through forced hospitalization and forced medication. Coercion is problematic because it erodes the rights of persons as responsible subjects.

Nevertheless, something else must be added to the argument set forth here about coercion. Here we foreground Tännsjö's argument, so that even when a person's autonomy is violated it is necessary to allow them to raise their concerns in forums that can challenge psychiatrization. To return to the powerful argument from hooks, it is important to foreground the *voice* of the person suffering with mental distress. This means fostering the hearing of voice in community—their own interpretation of their experience rather than another's interpretation, as well as challenging the systems that make the hearing of voice impossible.

For instance, understanding how gender and religiosity play a role together in psychiatric oppression, it is important to realize that women have, for several centuries, been penalized for speaking with their own authority. Specifically, speaking about God authoritatively and decisively has often been punished in legal and psychiatric fashion.[106] This understanding about the history of overlapping oppressions exerted by psychiatry and patriarchy helps us listen to the voices of people suffering from mental distress differently.

There are some helpful ways to give people more control over their psychiatric treatment. As we have seen, it is important to emphasize persons' freedom when possible. In addition to cultural awareness of the history of oppression, it is crucial to note the significance of psychiatric advanced directives (PADs) as tools that can be used so that a patient can have more autonomy over their medical decisions. These documents, in which an individual, "certified to be competent at the time, makes clear statements about preferences regarding treatment conditions to be preferred or avoided when they are next hospitalized."[107] On a psychiatric advanced directive form, a patient may state that they do not wish to be given neuroleptic medication or shock treatments. The contents of one's PAD can then be shared with close friends and family and with doctors and medical staff upon admission to a psychiatric facility. Some advocates offer training to certify persons to educate about these advanced directives, and have offered guidelines with which to use them.[108]

There are signs that PADs are desirable yet underutilized. A broad study by Peter Statsny discovered that although 73 percent of people wanted PADs, only seven percent had completed them.[109] "Patients were more likely to want an advanced directive if they were female, were of a racial or ethnic minority, had a history of self-harm, were under heavy external pressure to take medications, had police involved in a prior crisis, and had a low level of personal autonomy or mastery."[110] As such, the already marginalized sought more control over their psychiatric care. Most forms for PADs include spaces in which to place what kind of medication one wants and does not want, but no spaces to signal that one does not want to be treated with medication. Making PADs, and other similar tools, available to persons in communities and helping them choose their treatment preferences are significant steps toward full autonomy and independence, an ethical goal in the ethical treatment of people diagnosed with mental illness.

Intersectional Issues: Social Class and Psychiatry

In an article coauthored with a group of scholars at Boston University, Judi Chamberlin found that the single most important factor in whether c/s/x advocacy was helpful to persons was whether or not they had financial resources.[111] Canadian activist and educator David Reville argues that the new political activism of the c/s/x movement transformed the old psychiatric system of a "bed, a pill, and a rest," to a "home, a job, and a friend."[112] By reclaiming voice from the psy-system of treatment and coercion, c/s/x activists began asking that other aspects of their lives begin to be addressed. As such, discussing only self-definition issues will not be adequate unless the conditions for self-determination are also fostered. As noted in the *Strategies for Living* study cited previously, money was listed as an important concern for many c/s/x activists. Persons with mental diagnosis are more often poor, but poverty also contributes to mental distress, leading to an important intersection of oppressions and thus also a grounds for fostering solidarity.

As noted, the c/s/x critique does not simply travel in one direction but can also provide the basis for a critique of the neoliberal project of self-definition as a whole. In this way it offers provocative and helpful point of entry into economic analysis.

In the United Kingdom, a group of social workers found solidarity with psychiatric survivors in their argument for better rights for workers. During the strike, the survivors "entered and occupied one of the vacant premises... and were supported by the striking workers with food parcels and moral support."[113] In another instance, survivors fought for the reinstatement of a nurse who was fired for whistleblowing about the removal of services. Sometimes these initiatives engaged in multiple forms of intersection with the mental health system, even "occur[ing] *in defense* of particular mental health services."[114] After organizing for their own rights, a group of Harvard service workers turned to the nearby hospital with the slogan, "Pro-Patient, Pro-Union."[115] Again, it is worth emphasizing that these c/s/x activists were organizing *for* actual services, rather than against institutional control, since mental health care had been severely cut in their communities.

There are many paradoxes workers in psychiatric institutions and c/s/x activists face as they seek to build "deeply engaged relationships": workers may not be trusted because they represent the system and survivors might not be trusted because of a mentalism that still exists within the working class. Yet these paradoxes do not have to be simple contradiction but can lead to more meaningful engagements. It would also be interesting to understand how many of the service workers were themselves users of psychiatry. This intersectional focus builds on the early mad liberation emphasis, whose *Mad Network News* was published by union activists. One of the most important tension points is the tension over psychiatric knowledge; for example, after organizing and striking some c/s/x activists critiqued the framework for mental health care since they were as able union organizers as the supposedly sane.

Reaching such engagements becomes more feasible when workers and survivors recognize their shared fate and their shared oppression, simultaneously grappling with the fundamental imbalance of power. Since each group has many members who have been stigmatized by the multiple intersections of social oppression found in poverty, these groups have suffered in ways that could potentially draw them together during this neoliberal era.

Likewise, since each seek meaningful employment and a living wage, working together on economic projects becomes one way to think of preventative care for mental distress. Given the importance of poverty as a cause that leads to mental distress, as described in the first chapter, I argue that that such shared organizing can be helpful. For persons who have come in contact with the mental health system, the possibility of stigma means that they are chronically disempowered when it comes to organizing.

In order to move to some sort of relationship, this means confronting the bias that c/s/x survivors sometimes have against the state. Although it is an understandable bias, the c/s/x movement has engaged in skepticism about the state as a form of total control and this skepticism can play into a neoliberal framework where persons are expected to be able to foster their own mental well-being. As we saw in our last chapter, the fact of deinstitutionalization and the broken promises of the state for mental health care in the community meant that there were less services available for c/s/x advocates in the community. This fits into a logic of deinstitutionalization where people are expected to be responsible for themselves.

> Neoliberalism... seeks to claw back the gains of the welfare state under the ideological banner of "responsibility," "self-care," and "recovery." Examples of self-organization can all to readily be used as an excuse to reduce welfare services in the name of combating the so-called "welfare dependency culture."[116]

Resisting the tendency toward privatization in neoliberal economies while at the same time holding out the hope of more creative and innovative treatment methods, persons acting for solidarity can join forces. The banner of joint oppression, in which those suffering from economic exploitation are rendered vulnerable to mental distress, is one way that such activism can take place.

On the other hand, survivors of psychiatric treatment also must be able to see the "challenges faced by mental health workers" on their own terms and how access to care is also an important goal for activism in some communities. This is a challenge for the c/s/x movement because it has sometimes neglected its own roots in social-class activism, a form of consciousness-raising that continues to be crucial and at stake in challenging the laissez-faire politics of a neoliberal era.

The social model of disability described earlier in the chapter, which laid an emphasis on the social barriers to access rather than impairments, was actually developed by a group of socialist disability theorists: *The Union of the Physically Impaired against Segregation*. It is helpful to briefly explore the links between Marxist analysis and disability theorizing.

In some ways the concept of disability is a creation of the capitalist order, since it was only in the Industrial Revolution that differently abled persons were separated from family units of production and expected to create. Marxist theorists such as Roddy Slorach have argued that a competitive and capitalist culture in which one's value is consistently measured by one's input to the economy creates the conditions in which persons with disabilities have prejudice exercised against them and are socially excluded. Slorach imagines labor organizing as providing the basis for new solidarity between social classes, an approach that could lead persons across the disability spectrum to greater rights and participation, in Marx's phrase, "from each according to his abilities, to each according to his needs."[117] Since work is so often a matter of survival in practical as well as psychological terms, attending to the necessity and opportunity for work becomes a central concern for c/s/x activism.

Slorach notes how persons with physical disabilities have rejected those with mental illness as fitting into the category of disability, an approach which c/s/x activists have applauded by also excluding themselves from this category. Therefore, the challenge of the new psychiatric activism, if it is to combine intersectional concerns facing the c/s/x movement, it must agitate broadly for class and housing rights as well as making common cause with working-class concerns— the very workers within the psychiatric system who are also the most oppressed by it. Keeping in mind some of the central themes of this book—that widespread economic deprivation has led to conditions in which people experience more mental distress than ever before—means perceiving directly how economic oppression adds injury to injury by creating disability for persons who had already experienced a degree of economic exclusion. This does not mean that c/s/x activists abandon their concern for civil liberties and self-definition, but that this self-definition agenda can be linked to a broader project that also helps make self-determination possible. Understanding how working-class persons and c/s/x activists are marginalized and how their oppressions are linked can lead to shared solidarity between each group.

Becoming Partners to C/S/X Testimony

In a UK conference, a group of psychiatric survivors gathered to redefine self-harm as an act of survival from traumatic abuse rather than a suicide attempt or a sign of underlying pathology. Through the conference and the book that resulted, survivors began to challenge the prevalent psychiatric orthodoxy about self-harm and also invited outsiders to be changed by their stories:

> I'm Maggy and I started to cut my body 5 years ago. I go to casualty and get hauled onto the psychiatric bandwagon. I am then given a nice little "label." The current label is Schizophrenia... But how do I see myself? I am a survivor of sexual abuse and a survivor of the system... When I feel I am losing control, I reach for a razor to prove to myself that I can have control over my body. When I am lost for words, my cuts speak for me. They say—look—this is how much I am hurting inside. Self-injury... is not attention seeking. It is not a suicide attempt. It is a silent scream.[118]

In a recent article Mark Cresswell examines what it means to hear this kind of testimony and how it makes one into something more than an outside observer. At the same time, it does not mean that one has not gone through the experience oneself. Cresswell accesses the philosophical survivorship literature from the Holocaust, including voices such as Shosanna Felman, Dori Laub, and Giorgio Agamben, and he underscores the eventfulness of the kind of testimony that c/s/x advocates create through their movement. According to Agamben's distinction between two kinds of testimony, *testis*, in which one is the third party witness between two rivals, and *superstes*, "in which has lived through something from beginning to end and can therefore bear witness to it," c/s/x advocates would be like the latter kind of witness.[119] Making a third category, Cresswell argues that we can become partners when we hear c/s/x advocates.

This third category implies a social transformation has occurred through the event of bearing witness.[120] In order for this to occur one has to be changed by the event of testimony. There is always the possibility that the person testifying will not be believed or that her claims will be rejected. The claims of the self-harm conference were, for example, that self-harm did not imply psychiatric disorder and that is was concerned as much with self-preservation as with suicide. "The impact is affective, but also visceral, and not just cognitive. It is not the same as...the presentation of third person events."[121] In an executive summary published afterward, it was described as "one of the most *upsetting* and also encouraging events with which recipients have been involved in the last four or five years. The personal contributions from people who self-harm were *devastating*."[122]

The potential for being a partner to persons who have been diagnosed with mental illness involves the work of listening to their testimony about their experience and not remaining neutral in the face of it, but rather allowing it to move one to action. As we have seen, hearing someone's self-definition is crucial to fostering their dignity. At the same time, it means allowing one's full social world to enter into the picture. For example, in the self-harm conference, participants discussed the politics of gender and the significant role that trauma played. Becoming partners rather than passive spectators, people find their own stories profoundly shaped by the testimony of those whom they hear.

Understanding one's self as a witness implies ethical and legal responsibility as well as a sense of mutual entailment.[123] As we can see, with circumstances such as self-harm there can be profound ethical deliberations that caregivers make. The self-harm conference and the literature published from it orients professionals to protect the autonomy of harmers as much as possible and to give the harmers' voices priority.[124] It also helps them learn how to actively cope with the harming, thus beginning to take some control over it.

Cresswell maintains that becoming a partner means that you can accompany stories you have not been through, under the condition that you safeguard the integrity of the other's narrative. This is a significant point and must remain a central aspect of preserving voice for people who have been psychiatrized. We should not seek to overrun the voices of c/s/x survivors themselves through the category of partnership.

At the same time, given the wide range of emotional suffering in our time caused by financial pressures and the impact that these changes have on all persons in the working and contingent classes—who are an increasing portion of our society—then there is a widespread social suffering that persons are able to become partners with because they are able to imaginatively enter that suffering because of shared solidarity.

Emotional distress is always intersectional. By fostering c/s/x activism early union organizers supported MNN. Later on, survivors advocated for the rights of psychiatric service workers. Intersectional oppression means that persons diagnosed with mental illness are more likely to be in the contingent class and thus in more need of economic advocacy. Being positioned as witnesses to the widespread suffering of the neoliberal economy means opening our eyes to the inequality surrounding us, noting how it has caused many types of trauma and disintegration, and refusing to blame this suffering on individualistic causes in the brain or genes of particular persons. Mapping such social suffering means becoming a partner to testimony rather than neutrally observing it from a distance.

Ministers and counselors play this important role as partners in their communities. When they are not responsible to render a medical diagnosis, they have a unique opportunity to witness what people have been going through and engage a broader imagination for persons' stories. They may not have gone through the same suffering a given congregant has gone through, but they can partner with his concerns by showing solidarity. This broader imagination includes the testimony of faith and the capacity to bind people together in community. Sometimes it is faith itself which challenges an exclusively biomedical vision of the human person.

One of the parishioners at my local congregation has been in contact with the mental health system and has been in advocacy around the state, speaking to psychiatrists about informed consent for medication. This individual has worked to have a memorial erected at a local mental hospital where thousands of people were buried in a mass grave. He has allowed me to use his story without using his name, so we will call him Jim. He has positioned me as a partner by describing his more than 160 shock treatments, given by a doctor who claimed to know simply by looking at him whether he needed shock treatments.

Jim discusses hospitality among religious communities frequently, noting how important early involvement with a Quaker retreat was in his own formation. He also discusses the importance of work: in his early life a clergy person gave him the job of sexton at his church after only meeting him once, giving him the keys to the church. Indeed, it is his decades-long involvement with local congregations that has made him feel that his entire experience of suffering and creativity that he has endured through psychotic breaks has been worthwhile. He says that it has taken him more than 30 years to come to this conclusion.

He came up with his own diagnosis, which he wrote up in pamphlets that he has distributed to his psychiatrist, social worker, and to me:

> I've finally come to a conclusion that accurately encapsulates my disorder... I now know that I've been afflicted with "inverse paranoia"—the belief that people and the world are out to do me good—this disorder has caused me to reach out to a wide diversity of people and it has caused me to see the good in others... I intend to combat and overcome this disorder in the year ahead by reading [a conservative local newspaper] everyday as well as watching two hours of Fox cable news—hoard my money and personal possessions and when anyone smiles at me, say inwardly to myself "What's he up to?"[125]

Returning the diagnosis in ironic prose, Jim has shifted the conceptual category of mental illness and made me a partner to his testimony in the process. During a recent hospitalization his pastor and another parishioner sought to bring him communion in the mental hospital, but they were denied the ability to bring in any food or drink, so the religious elements of communion had to be left behind in a visitors locker. They came on to the ward, after emptying their pockets in front of the security guard, and stood just outside his door, since Jim was not receiving visitors at that time. Through the open doorway, they prayed aloud for him at the end of their visit. The psychiatric refusal of the body and blood of Christ did not prohibit communion from happening, although it did interfere with one of the sacred acts of the faith.

Afterward, talking with the pastor about his hospitalization, Jim described how he had felt depersonalized in the mental hospital. The pastor did not bring up the subject of his hospitalization herself, but waited until he talked about it. "Did you see that?" Jim asked. "Did you see how they had just a little slot where they could dispense medication? Like at a gas station? Did you see how impersonal that was?"

Consumer/survivor/ex-patient activism occurs in Christian communities around the nation as pastors hear the narratives of people who have come into contact with the psychiatric system. They listen to the person's own self-description. Do they understand themselves as patients—I am schizophrenic; as consumers—I am a user of mental health services because of schizophrenia, or are they survivors or ex-patients—I hear voices or used to hear voices? In attending to these stories, ministers and counselors attend to the body of Christ in their midst. In this sense, people diagnosed with mental illness are not outsiders who need charity, but rather persons who make up God's visible presence in our midst, deserving dignity and the best spiritual care, which demands the capacity for both self-definition and self-determination.

In becoming partners to the stories of the people with mental distress in their lives, ministers and counselors help to shape the individual's experience of suffering with mental distress. Looking beyond the mentalism and methodological individualism inherent in an exclusively biomedical model for mental illness, they are able to help interpret how social and economic suffering have caused harm that has contributed to psychic distress, for example, the conditions of capitalism in a situation where workers are oppressed or the conditions of racism in a racist society.

Rather than seeing the person in their care primarily as stricken by a disease that will run its inevitable course, the minister is in a position to ask questions about the experience of illness, for example, how the person has already tried to cope with phenomena related to mental distress such as hearing voices, or what types of social and emotional supports have been most helpful to the person. Since people with mental distress have stated that one of their most important needs is for a helping person to talk to about their problems,[126] ministers and counselors can offer this listening ear, provided they are conceptually attuned to see the person as more than an individual with a disordered brain, but as a person who is actively making sense of their experience.[127] It is important that, instead of fearing a person who suffers from mental distress, a minister or counselor move toward them with interest and compassion, listening to their own distinctive testimony.

CHAPTER 4

Pastoral Counseling and Social-Class Shame

Robert had been unemployed for some time and his discouragement made it necessary for him to seek a counselor. He came to a pastoral counselor because the counseling center used a sliding scale to make counseling more affordable. When he arrived late for the first appointment, his pastoral counselor Christina did not seem upset, but definitely noticed. He spent most of the first session talking about his discouragement and despair and his sense of life not adding up.

Delving into the conversation a little bit deeper, she discovered that he had lost his job when the factory closed down several years ago, and, after cycling through several jobs, felt chronic discouragement.[1] His marriage had crumbled, in large part because of financial stress, and he had begun drinking heavily in the process. Under all the pressure, his wife left with the children and began another home far away.

Robert kept describing himself as a "failure" and Christina came up empty with what to say. She had been watching programs on nightly news shows about the economy and knew that persons in his position were making less than they actually needed for housing and food by working at service jobs.[2] She was familiar with the critiques of income inequality.

Robert seemed to be aware of Christina's class. She noticed that he paid attention to her professional attire and the well-furnished office building where they met. By the end of the conversation she saw that he looked down and away.

Robert emphasized that he did not feel connected to anybody. She had noted that he seemed to be withdrawing even as they spoke and wondered if he would come back for another session. They had worked on some feasible goals, such as making a plan for addressing his drinking and exploring his story, but she had a sinking feeling that she could not quite put her finger on. She realized that she felt a nagging sense of guilt: her feeling of having too much and wondering what she could do to help. Perhaps on Robert's end there was a sense of shame that he felt for being poor. The phenomenon of shame is a complex emotional reality, and I explore how to work with shame in my analysis of a psychology of poverty shame. This is a seldom-explored aspect of shame.[3]

Addressing shame requires explicitly working through social class and the effects of poverty. Research has shown that counselees want issues of social class to be addressed in counseling—and indeed the entire therapeutic alliance is at stake in addressing these concerns.[4] In Christina's therapeutic relationship with Robert, she is likely to make stereotypical comments that indicate she does not understand what he has to do to survive. She may even treat his mental suffering as a reality separate from his economic struggles. Nevertheless, she does not need to just become more *understanding* of the differences between them in order to become a better pastoral counselor—she also needs to advocate for Robert in order to change the conditions that *take labo*r from Robert unfairly. As such, a recognition paradigm alone is unable to deal with social class, but there must be a way to help a client ameliorate the difficult position that he is in. Social-class conversation is not merely consciousness-raising, but it is also transformative.

In this chapter I explore pastoral counseling in the new economy as something that can transform both the feelings associated with and practical conditions of being in the working-class position. The context of counseling is well suited to interpret an experience that involves both psychic pain and the need for solutions.

In previous chapters we have explored how current categories for mental health and mental illness are profoundly shaped by economic suffering. When we individualize this suffering, however, and describe it exclusively in the language of the medical model, we lose some of the nuances of social class, mistaking psychological suffering as its primary cause for financial difficulties when in fact it is often an effect of it.

There is always the possibility that power can be used against working-class clients and so caution must be exercised to safeguard these relationships. Mental health users frequently speak about the cross-class relationships that they have with medical professionals, which include these professionals keeping private diagnostic notes on clients, holding case conferences about clients without their knowledge, and cooperating with state agencies without disclosing to clients. If there is already the potential for mistrust in a cross-class relationship, these practices may only deepen it.

Understanding and ameliorating social-class shame requires both indirect and sometimes, direct means for working with shame. Socially engaged psychology can be useful for resisting the shame that comes from impoverishment. This can include challenging the idea that it is the fault of working-class people that they are poor. Robert may feel like a failure, but understanding economic changes in the last several decades helped Christina interpret Robert's suffering more broadly with him. Such psychology fosters accountability, transparency, and thereby empowerment. This chapter offers several examples of this approach to psychology, including group work that discusses the effects of poverty.

Christina considered herself a minister in the broadest sense and described herself as a pastoral counselor. For her, this meant that she sought to help clients with spiritual concerns, assist them to talk about their problems and find support, and also believe that a person's faith was too important to be ignored in counseling. She described her approach to counseling as fostering the *dignity* and *empowerment* of clients.

Christina considered her clients to be persons created in the Image of God and thereby worth dignity and respect. She prayed for them between sessions. Her theological commitments entered into her counseling as they framed how she helped people through their trials but she did not necessarily bring up her faith with clients. She thought of her work as helping people live meaningfully, a task inspired and sustained by her faith, which served to support what she did as a pastoral counselor, even though she was not officially ordained.

Some pastoral theologians have argued that pastoral counselors also use a type of diagnosis that is inherently theological.[5] I submit that a theological framework for interpreting a person's life is essential. When Christina considers Robert's situation, she keeps in mind two aspects of the human person—how a person is created in the Image of God with inherent dignity, worth, and purpose, including a particular vocation for the individual's life. Helping working-class clients find their double voice (both dignity and vocation) requires pastoral sensitivity and something further. In order to offer this kind of theological perspective, pastoral counselors must be firmly rooted in the very material concerns of clients' everyday life. This means that they must be as concerned about housing and transportation as they are about family systems and interpersonal relationships.

Pastoral counseling, a specialist approach that addresses the religious and spiritual concerns of persons who are suffering from psychic distress, is in some ways a perfect place to examine how the theoretical material in the first three chapters comes to life and is transformed by practice. It might seem that pastoral counseling is closer to the *psy-complex* because of its clinical nature, yet bringing dignity to persons and helping them find their vocation are significant aims of both counseling and ministry approaches to care. The tools that we can use to foster a pastoral counseling approach include a public psychology that turns toward the outer world in order to transform it.

As a therapist, Christina has asked Robert to fill out intake forms and now has the challenge of developing a DSM diagnosis. She looks through her options—anxiety, depression, and substance abuse—but discovers not one of them matches exactly what she has experienced with Robert. I might suggest that a more appropriate social diagnosis may be isolation secondary to embarrassment, since Robert has lost significant relationships because of poverty and this is impacting his psychic functioning.[6]

However she uses that information, she also has the challenge of reading the signs of our times, namely the wider factors that contribute to social suffering and distress. Reading the community's pain is as important as reading one person's diagnostic chart. Understanding the interlocking relationship between person and community means that no approach is adequate unless it unites the two.

In order for Christina to keep Robert as a client she will need to show both understanding and a realistic sensitivity in addressing the dynamics of class. Indeed, many counseling relationships are *cross-class* relationships, with the counselor in the professional class and the client in the working or contingent class. In order to approach counseling as a cross-class relationship, it is important to both deconstruct commonly held notions of poverty and construct positive shared knowledge about what it means to be in a particular class position. It will also mean thinking beyond the 50-minute-hour to address the social circumstances that are contributing to Robert's poverty and thus to his life being so difficult from day to day, thereby engaging in some form of advocacy. Counselors are frequently in a *contradictory class location* to their working-class clients, meaning that they are more likely to make alliances with upper-class persons to shore up their own social-class position. This can cause a counselor to miss many aspects of a client's life.

A participant in a social counseling group discussing depression described her working-class experience:

> Middle-class women don't pay for their groceries with food stamps and WIC vouchers, they don't pay their rent with Section 8, or micromanage a myriad of ongoing appointments with various social service agencies

and programs that are there to support you, but only if you beg just a little. They don't glean other people's scraps collecting food boxes when their food stamps don't last until the end of the month. They don't know the humiliation and self-belittlement involved in going to these offices to ask their agents for help, being treated like dirt in their offices, and then returning to the world to be treated like dirt again when offering the vouchers you had to grovel for in exchange for goods and services.[7]

In order to live their way into a different world from their own, counselors need to develop critical distance from their own taken-for-granted class assumptions, a process that requires becoming a partner to stories quite different from their own narrative.

Addressing social class in a nuanced way is helpfully done by engaging in both deconstructive elements and constructive elements. Deconstructive elements involve challenging stereotypes that posit an individualistic cause for poverty and thus describe a working-class person as a "type." Yet there are also constructive elements to social-class counseling. Persons who understand class as an interdependent set of relationships between workers and owners can ask about the conditions under which one has to work, exploring the effects of daily working conditions on physical and psychic well-being and spirituality. Here the goal is transformation—ameliorating what is oppressive about these relationships and changing them. Pastoral counselors, by the very nature of their vocation, wish to preserve the dignity of their clients, attending to both the Image of God and human purposefulness in each narrative, rather than treating a person's story in utilitarian or fiscal terms.

I suggest that Christina must think differently about the efficacy of counseling when she counsels Robert. In the past she has frequently thought that it is empathy that heals. Simply by becoming attuned to the experience of another she could imagine her way into his experience, thus creating validation for him that would be healing. In order for pastoral counseling with working-class persons to be effective, solidarity must be added to empathy.[8]

Empathy is one significant step: As liberation theologian Joerg Rieger argues, "We need to take a closer look at what difference religion makes for those who experience the logic of downturn in their own bodies."[9] Empathy helps us understand how the downturn has affected those in working-class positions, but it is only a first step.

Solidarity means being willing to take risks for advocacy and empowerment and it suggests that there are additional goods beyond just individual empowerment that are in view. Offering a cross-class relationship that focuses on flourishing of the person in all areas and which highlights the voice of the other, underscoring their own self-definition, pastoral counseling needs to more consciously use its power. In order for solidarity to be effective, it has to transform both parties.

In this chapter I attempt to persuade counselors to directly address social class along with mental distress. Theological issues are at stake. I am convinced that we must care more about pastoral counseling for the working class rather than simply diagnosis and treatment through psychiatric terms—this means valuing persons as having dignity and a vocation and expressing this in therapeutic conversation. Persons in the working class are often medicated more heavily than wealthier persons and have less access to psychotherapy or counseling.[10] Likewise, people who have been diagnosed with mental illness increasingly receive medication instead of therapy, which may lead them to feel better but may not allow their voice to be heard.

I argue that *pastoral counseling*, conceived of as a site of resistance that addresses the misplaced shame of a neoliberal economy, is a helpful and transformative resource for persons suffering from emotional distress since it helps them discover dignity and vocation and assists them to reclaim their voice, without which solidarity is ineffective.

Behind the term "pastoral counseling" is the official discipline and its guild—the Association of Pastoral Counselors (AAPC)—which began in 1963 and proliferated through a set of counseling centers.[11] By understanding pastoral counseling and its history, I maintain that it is important to reclaim something that has been lost in the tradition, namely the century-old voice of the Social Gospel as a basis for pastoral counseling.[12] Building on this tradition can be done in a variety of clinical spaces. I have in mind the broader set of counselors who are inspired by religious and spiritual concerns and see faith as a context for their psychotherapeutic work with clients.

The Relationship of Pastoral Counseling as Interpretive

Pastoral counseling is an interpretive relationship that begins with a story. Describing how pastoral counseling is different from pastoral care, Donald Capps argues that "in [pastoral counseling], we *are* asking for something more than a listening ear and a word of assurance. We want the pastor to join with us in interpreting the story we tell, and we hope that the pastor, by virtue of her training and experience, will be able to see things in the story that we cannot see."[13] Note the element of invitation and the implicit structure in this relationship. The fact that this is a more formal relationship facilitates a trust that allows counselors to be more forthright in helping persons interpret the social factors impinging upon them. Recent efforts in the pastoral counseling literature have begun to discuss the impact of oppression on the human psyche and how pastoral counselors must take a different role in helping persons interpret this anxiety.

For one, Carroll Watkins-Ali in her book *Survival and Liberation: Pastoral Theology in African American Context* describes her work with African American women suffering from the oppression of "genocidal poverty."[14] She addresses the multiple oppressions these women face by helping them get grants to pay for therapy and also advocating for them in cultural spaces such as schools to get the access that they need. Speaking in the African American context, she underscores how discriminatory housing policies have kept this community poor but how counseling helps them find support through the experience of children's disability and violent child bereavement.[15] She reorients the field away from a model of empathy alone toward one of advocacy and empowerment, in which the well-being of the entire community is in the foreground. Many of the changes facing African American communities have also been felt by poor and working-class whites in recent years, so that including a more explicitly social-class component helps explain significant aspects of this suffering. Much of what she said about poverty also applies in poor communities in rural areas, for example.[16]

Additionally, in a recent book Kirk Bingaman focuses on the "core theological beliefs" that sustain people through what he calls the new American "age of anxiety."[17] He gives examples of counselors offering theological reassurances to clients too easily. He notes how uncomfortable people are talking about religious beliefs even though faith is crucially important to many Americans. Because he repeatedly refers to economic realities, Bingaman's notion of anxiety is not generalized, but related to specific economic factors of our time, namely the changes related to neoliberalism.

Yet his book lacks an analysis of social class, one of the most significant factors contributing to the new anxiety for persons. Likewise, the reliance on cognitive schemas (negative thoughts that impact one's behaviour), may risk denying the very real and complex oppressions that are reasonable stressors in a person's life.

Though each of these recent works refers to economic suffering, more could be done to bring it to the foreground in the counseling context. The goal of pastoral counseling is to make explicit the contextual factors that persist in the background of someone's therapeutic conversation in order to more intentionally interact with them. Pastoral counselors are becoming increasingly adept at talking about race and culture with their clients—the AAPC has guidelines for this on its website—yet there is no mention of how to discuss social class or why it is important to do so.[18] Misunderstanding, and even injustice, is likely in such a relationship unless social class becomes an explicit part of the conversation.

Lauren Marie Appio studied the experience of working-class persons in psychotherapy and demonstrated that working-class persons who have gone to see counselors want their counselors to directly address issues pertaining to class and, unless they do so, counselors put the therapeutic relationship in jeopardy.[19] She recommended that counselors "assess whether clients are able to meet their basic needs for housing, clothing, food, and healthcare."[20] If counselors did not address such concerns, and if they did not feel comfortable talking about the material realities in clients' lives, clients began to regard them as untrustworthy and began keeping important information from the counselors.

Working-class participants in Appio's study talked about times that counselors exhibited something akin to microaggressions, suggesting solutions for client's problems without realizing the obstacles that may be in the way (e.g., "Why don't you just go back to school?"). Microaggressions are unconscious verbal assaults that are prejudicial and have the effect of othering a person. When the counselor begins having stereotypes of working-class clients play through her mind, it becomes part of a "social class countertransference," a story the counselor is telling herself about the client related to her preconceived notions about class.[21] When a counsellor is using social class countertransference, she is more likely to engage in microaggressions. Instead of these stereotypical responses, working-class clients need a chance for both advocacy and reinterpretation.

On the one hand, some counselees express visible frustration in counselors who have little to offer in terms of helping with their practical needs such as housing. This indicates to a counselee that their counselor may not be the most adept at interpreting the suffering stemming from chronic unemployment, the despair over debt, the dilemmas of foreclosure, and other pressing everyday stressors. So one part needs to be advocacy in which the counselor has resources at hand.

On the other hand, when counselors can help clients interpret their difficulties not simply as their own fault, but as a part of an entire society of impoverishment and inequity, then a counselor is more likely to help persons resist the internal attribution of blame for something that is quite often the result of social suffering. This is how pastoral counselors can use the power of *discourse,* defined in chapter 2, to assist clients. In order to foster a pastoral counseling alliance with a client, it is necessary to address issues pertaining to social class in more than a cursory fashion.

If indeed pastoral counseling is an interpretive relationship in which the pastor is expected to know something to help the client make sense of their experience, and if the role of economic suffering is profound enough to shape the mental distress that persons face in the neoliberal era, then pastoral counseling without social-class analysis fails to completely interpret person's difficulties. Some pastoral counselors may object and state that this puts pastoral counselors more in the position of social workers, with whom they could consult, yet I argue that such a holistic approach to seeing someone's life is crucial in order to avoid both misunderstanding and injustice from occurring. From a relational perspective, economics and finances are simply too important to a person's sense of themselves to remain a footnote to pastoral counseling.

When Robert described to Christina how he was a "failure," she immediately started thinking about a recent news program she had seen in which persons in Milwaukee described themselves as "failures" after the factory had closed and they went to find work in the service sector.[22] *When he came back for counseling, she had taped a graph on the wall that described the extent of income inequity and another (figure 1.1) that showed the extent of the new working class. Robert took a close look at each of the graphs as he sat down. "Man, I should have guessed it was that bad," he said, as he sat down. "I'm glad you put that up there."*

Social-Class Inquiry as a Crucial Moment of Interpretation

In the second session Robert described some of his work experiences to Christina and she asked him follow-up questions. He discussed being out looking for work this week, riding on his bicycle from store to store, and noted how people seemed to treat him with contempt. As she was listening to him, she started thinking about her own debt, and how difficult it was for her to make it through college, and how she only managed to go to graduate school because of an extensive grant package. Looking at the debt bills now when they came in the mail immediately made her nauseated. When he finished speaking, she realized that he was the third person she spoke with this week that was struggling with unemployment: Why weren't these people talking with one another?

In this pastoral counseling conversation about social class, Christina is not looking for the expression of painful feeling for its own sake, as in the notion of catharsis, but hoping to link her client to the right sources of support, developing the kinds of relationships that can sustain him and transform society. It is not enough to simply know about class: we must be actively committed to more egalitarian relationships even as we engage in these conversations. Rather than taking social arrangements for granted, it is important to work for a society that has less marked social-class differentials.

She asked him, "What is one thing that you remember most clearly about your time working?" and Robert told her a story about a job he had gotten briefly after the factory closed as a maintenance worker at a nearby motel and how a customer had insulted him and spit on his shoe. He talked about the boiling rage that he felt, the deep humiliation, and how he coped with that humiliation to make it through work that day without striking the customer. He knew his manager would not be helpful. "Yet something twisted inside me that day. Something I don't know if I'll ever get back." Robert's traumatic memory is not remarkable because it stands alone, but is striking because these things happen to working-class persons everyday.

The social-class theory described in chapter 1 indicated that hierarchical statuses that are split out like layers on a cake miss some significant aspects about class. We should not depend upon a simple gradient approach that measures income or education to see how society is stratified. These approaches do not measure wealth, which has a much more enduring effect on social class than income alone.[23] Yet more fundamentally, they do not show the relational nature of class. This aspect indicates that class is made up of owners and workers and that each group needs each other. It is significant to explore the in-between position of managers and professionals who have authority or credentials to sell on the marketplace.

Robert's class position is defined by being working class. This means having to sell one's labor on the marketplace without owning the means of production. Pastoral counseling that addresses social class must explore what it means to be in this position—to have your body as your only tool for work, not for your own self or your family, but from which someone else can extract labor.

This relational nature of social class is a significant way to address how widespread economic factors impact individual persons. *Macro-social* arrangements have to do with the movement of global capital, such as neoliberalism's effect on entire nations as privatized entities and globalized working class. *Micro-social* arrangements have to do with the impact of these macro-factors on an individual's life and relationships. Understanding social class helps us see how *micro* processes are expressions of *macro* processes and how these small-level processes foster broader injustice.

The *micro* realities of social class have to do with two things. First, "What you *have* determines what you get."[24] This has to do with how "rights and powers people have over productive assets ... are a systematic determinant of standard of living."[25] *When Christine asked Robert what was the biggest impediment to him getting a good paying job, he stated, "lacking reliable transportation."* This meant that his housing had to be near work and thus it limited his options for work. Since social class helps determine assets, it also helps determine chances that come from these resources. Understanding this principle means that the systemic factors of working-class reality include much more than simply income: they involve housing, transportation, and access to various social goods.

The impact of class on a person's opportunities can be explored with pastoral counseling inquiry. Some questions that explore this first point include, "What is your daily routine like?" "If your car broke down and you had to have it fixed, how would you get to work?" and "If someone had a different starting place than you had, how would their work be different from the kind of work you have to do?" Asking such questions is different than asking about income—a major taboo in US society—but instead involves asking about the conditions in which one starts off, whether with many resources or with the deck stacked against them.

The second point is that "What you *have* determines what you *have to do to get what you get.*"[26] This means that your income, wealth, and social connections impact the kind of work you will have to do to survive. Some questions a pastoral counselor could ask to explore this point include, "What do you have to do to make ends meet? Has your employer ever made you do something against your principles? How did they do it? What do you wish you could show a rich person about your day—give them a snapshot?" This final question does not simply instigate class struggle, since that struggle already exists—for example, workers struggle to get paid and owners struggle to get their workers to work for less pay. Rather, this final question allows for an important reversal—since we are bombarded by images of exorbitant wealth, this line of questioning allows the client to discuss painful and chronic stressors in their life.

The example of Robert's shoe being spit upon in the previous vignette was a case of this—he had to simply manage that experience and move on, continuing to face potential disgrace, in order to work and hopefully pay rent for the next month. Seemingly, this point directly relates to labor, namely Robert has to make multiple applications at low-wage service jobs. Yet this point also leads to questions of power and rights, namely how employers at these jobs can ask him psychological questions on their application forms, or ask him to give urine samples without privacy,[27] or search his possessions on the job, all within their legal rights.

These questions and others like it should be part of the intake of clients, since a person's life includes their dignity and purpose at work as much as it includes their family and interpersonal relationships and their spiritual faith. Counselors should show as much interest in these factors as they do in family-of-origin dynamics and internal object relations. Such questions put a mirror up to the experience of social class and help the counselor and client interpret the distress that arises from being in a working-class position differently from simply through psychiatric frameworks. Neglecting what it means to work is tantamount to neglecting a chief source of stress, anxiety, and meaning in people's lives.

Rather than being invasive, such questions build understanding and help people feel less alone. Working-class clients say that they want a counselor to see their "standard of living, working conditions, level of toil, leisure, material security."[28] Some may worry if these questions offend, but they actually come as a relief.

Not only do class questions help clients feel less alone, but they also help working- class clients becoming aware of their interests. Once they understand that they are not alone but belong to a class formation that has power, they can struggle for what they need with others in a similar position. Despite the fact that workers have been pitted against each other, laborers across races and ethnicities and even across national borders have more in common with each other than they have with owners.[29] Beginning to feel less alone is a step along the way to learning strategies for challenging working-class marginalization, exploring "the strategies of individual workers within the labor process to reduce their level of toil, to conflicts between highly organized collectivities of workers and capitalists over the distribution of rights and powers within production."[30] This could be called strategic counseling that focuses on the conditions of work. The hopeful outcome of this process is that people will realize that there are others who are going through similar types of struggles and that they will organize with others to help alleviate the conditions that lead to such unnecessary suffering.

Some questions that help clients develop such a relationship include, "When have you seen a fellow worker do something to get treated more fairly at work?" and "What would that company you worked at have done if all the sudden all the workers refused to come in to work?" "Have you ever done something management wouldn't like to help a fellow worker to be better off?"

Such questions help clients to explore the relational nature of social class. Not only does Robert have to sell his labor to be working class, but also owning class persons have to utilize his labor in order to make their stores and businesses run, so being in a certain social class is always a relational experience. This is simply one kind of relationship that has yet to be addressed adequately in pastoral counseling. There are multiple pressures on the job that make these kinds of conversations unlikely or impossible, and managers frequently interfere with privacy of workers to stop such conversations from happening. Pastoral counseling can be a site of resistance where such conversations can take place.

By the end of the discussion, Christina had asked several of these questions, and Robert had become more animated, thinking of a time when a friend had shared food with a pregnant maintenance worker and kept her from having to do a dangerous job. Note that these questions are not simply idealistic solutions that fall outside of the framework of labor, but involve looking for sites of resistance within the experience of working itself. We discuss the psychological significance of these questions in the next section.

Christina ended the session by giving Robert the name of a local group who worked on transportation issues for workers. Likewise, she gave him information about a forum that was discussing the relationship between poverty and emotional distress (this was happening at a local congregation) and that was engaging in advocacy to change these conditions. He said he might look into the latter in another circumstance, but he was just too busy trying to survive. The former opportunity seemed especially interesting to him.

Christina began to be convinced that she needed to address the circumstances that contributed to Robert's poverty and not simply care personally for his suffering through a traditional one-on-one counseling relationship. That night she contacted the local chapter of *Jobs with Justice* to contribute money. She noticed when their next meeting was and put it on her calendar. In attending one of their local rallies and listening to working-class narratives, she expanded her own stories about working-class experience, and in the process she is directly addressing her *social-class countertransference*. Social-class countertransference is the term for the counselor's stereotyped and narrow stories about class that they place upon the working-class client's experience.[31]

Christina is beginning to realize that she is in a *contradictory class location*, meaning that she has some elements of a working-class position but also some elements of an owner-class position. Christina works with the power of *discourse*, that is, the capacity to use language to name and define the range of people's suffering and thereby propose concrete actions to reduce that suffering. We return to talk about the complexities of this class location later in the chapter.

Pastoral Counselors Addressing the Shame of Poverty

Christina's primary task in a pastoral counseling relationship with Robert is to ensure his safety and well-being and also to help him become more able to thrive, both as a person of dignity and a person whose life has purpose. I have argued that a public psychology is necessary that grapples with the experience of being in the working class. This means that she must challenge the unnecessary shame that comes with the experience of poverty, a shame that is propped up by notions of individual personal responsibility and narratives of the American Dream.

Robert is likely to feel shame in his relationship with Christina unless social class is addressed in ways that resist shame. Since Robert has multiple experiences every day that may contribute to him feeling shamed, from averted eyes when he crosses the street to being forced to urinate in the presence of a welfare worker,[32] this resistance against shame will be a monumental task indeed. Paradoxically, avoiding undue shame in pastoral counseling concerning poverty means being willing to address shame.

The belief in a meritocracy that anyone can succeed in if they work hard enough underlines much American thought and contributes to the shaming of the poor, even though upward mobility is rare. As I explored in chapter 1, children's descriptions of the poor shifted as they were socialized to see the poor as having personality traits that led them into poverty. While Latinos and African Americans were more likely to see the working-class persons as suffering from structural factors, they were also likely to believe the owner class had earned their wealth, a fact which numerous studies describing inherited wealth have disproven.[33] There is no meritocracy, but instead social class remains quite stable in the US context. Citing Thomas Hertz, theologian Joerg Rieger notes that "children from low income families have only a one percent chance of reaching the top five percent of the income distribution, versus children of the rich who have about a twenty-two percent chance."[34]

If people do not have the same chances across class positions, why would they feel shame about poverty? Many cultures across the world have beliefs about wealth and poverty that do not match with economic realities and contribute to shame. As Oxford economist Robert Walker suggests in a multinational study of attitudes about poverty, "The expectation that adults should be able to make their way in the world and to provide and care for their children and families financially and in other ways is a universal and longstanding social norm that underpins economic production and social order."[35] Using a cross-cultural analysis, Walker goes so far as to say that shame may be a nearly universal aspect of poverty.

What may be a longstanding social norm is also reinforced in relationships of injustice. Managers deploy shame to keep their workers in line. In her telling journalistic exploration *Nickel and Dimed: On Not Getting By in America,* Barbara Ehrenreich described how she had attempted to make ends meet by working low-paying jobs as a waitress, a maid, and a Wal-Mart employee. She describes the social degradations that she experienced as a worker.[36] She narrated not being allowed to use the restroom during an eight-hour shift, having her purse searched by a manager, and multiple mandatory drug tests. She concluded that these activities were more about social control, namely, that they inculcated in the working-class persons the sense that they were a reprobate, a criminal, and had no rights. They reinforced shame. After only a short time being treated in this way, she describes how these sentiments had an effect on her personhood. She began to wonder if she was a trustworthy person and the insults that persons gave her stung and haunted her.

The Shame-Affect Bind

Social-class shame is the combination of the high promises of the American Dream and the low benefits that accrue to many workers, combined with the daily insults of working under management. Understanding this shame and grappling with its effects is a crucial part of an intentionally social-class approach to pastoral counseling.

Shame can be defined as an overweening self-consciousness that evaluates the self as somehow bad or faulty. An emotion of comparison, it can be clustered with humiliation and embarrassment. Walker's study suggested that poor people are often the targets of shame-based discourse that can, in turn, lead to further social stratification.[37] Shame as "an unpleasant emotion appertaining to the inner self that leads to concealment, retreat, avoidance, and ultimately to disintegration and even suicide" which Walker, drawing from Amartya Sen, describes as the "irreducible absolutist core" of the experience of poverty.[38] Shame has to do on the individual level with the need to spare oneself the psychic trauma of exposure under the gaze of another;[39] and on the social end it has to do with the specter of disgrace and humiliation.

On the one hand, it should be noted that shame is not bad in and of itself: in many societies it is an emotion that is used to foster group cohesion. Psychologist Gershen Kaufman suggested that shame was not an emotion to be avoided but rather with which to cope.[40] On the other hand, while shame seems to be intended as a form of coercive social behavior to return the individual to the group, it often has the opposite effect, with those facing shame becoming ever more isolated and more likely to engage in antisocial behavior.[41] In a powerful series of books on shame, he has written about how each of us make bids to have power in our relationships with one another and have our interpersonal needs met. When people use power over us to deny these needs, it creates a "shame/affect bind," namely the experience of shame comes to take the place of other feelings that could be felt, such as anger or sadness. The shame-affect bind comes to occur so frequently that it becomes the default mechanism. Whenever someone gets angry they suddenly switch to shame, seen in self-talk such as "I can't believe how stupid I am." One is only able to address shame-affect binds with a chance to speak authentically about shame. This allows one to release these other emotions by decoupling them from shame.

There are helpful instances of this approach in recent literature. For example, critiquing the biomedical model of depression, Rogers-Vaughn argued that to see depression exclusively as a brain disease whose symptom was chemical imbalance, when so many social factors were making it harder for persons to climb the social ladder or even earn a living wage was to increase the capacity for self-blame, with the result of "shame."[42] He notes that this may help explain why societies with greater inequality have more depression.[43] Exploring a compounding factor, he maintains that frequently "when the individual who sees herself as depressed feels responsible for her predicament and thus becomes more depressed."[44] A limited individualistic model of psychic suffering thus contributes to the experience of shame and must be deconstructed.

One way to do this is to begin to talk about the shame that is all too often associated with the experience of working-class identity, and thus directly address the phobic reaction to shame in American culture, what Kaufmann calls a "shame about shame."[45] Talking about class is one way of addressing the phobic avoidance of shame. In her book on racism, *Learning to be White,* Thandeka discusses how racism is often linked to the experience of social-class shame and why it is necessary to address this shame in order to work toward intersectional justice that alleviates racism and classism at the same time.[46] The conversational strategies described previously, chronicling the everyday trauma of working, is one step toward this process.

Shame is an emotion of comparison that contains valences of societal expectations. In a neoliberal era there is a strong pressure to succeed, to monetize one's self by becoming an entrepreneur, while at the same time there are less resources to achieve this purported success. Being working class today means being acutely aware of the extent of others' wealth. Media images bombard a person with suggestions of profound wealth even while one is barely making and surrounded by the signs of suffering within one's community. The idea that one should be able to measure up is a catalyst for shame.

People experience shame from poverty and attempt to defend against it by trying to keep up social relationships with those in their communities and this often involves spending unaffordable amounts to keep social obligations. In other cases people react to the threat of shame by withdrawing from others. Some experience anger at perceived shame through destructive behavior. Others turn to blaming scapegoats such as addicts or the mentally ill.[47]

Note that these are relational strategies, indicating that shame is fundamentally a reality that has to do with one's interpersonal and social world and with the image of oneself that is projected into the social world. Robert Walker notes that anger can be a response to the perceived shame of poverty and that this anger can be used to challenge the systems that contribute to poverty.[48] In order to release the shame-affect bind it is necessary to deconstruct notions of personal responsibility and conceive of working-class experience without shame.

Drawing from the work of Ming Yan, Walker argues that there are four possible realities at the intersection of shame and poverty, each of which is shaped by two factors.[49] One factor was whether a person has actually been shamed and another factor is whether the person feels shame. Obviously it was possible for a person to have been shamed and feel shame about their poverty and in this case both factors would have been present. On the other hand, it was possible—perhaps more often in societies other than the United States—that persons were not shamed for their poverty yet felt shame, perhaps because of a highly internalized sense of honor. It was also possible that a poor person could be neither shamed nor feel shame about their poverty, an ideal situation that might only come about as a result of widespread education about the effects of neoliberalism on the working poor in the twenty-first century. In this case no one would shame others for their poverty.

Walker offers a tantalizing possibility that has not been described in any of these options. It was also possible that a person was shamed—maybe others critiqued her for using WIC stamps at the checkout line—but that she did not feel shame about their poverty. This would be a situation in which the other was shaming you, but you didn't feel shame.

One route to this resistance is interpretive. Given what we have seen in the book thus far, it is important to emphasize that the widespread economic suffering of our times indicates that one need not feel ashamed about being in the working or contingent class since poverty from working class social position is a widespread reality in the United States. US pastoral counselors talking to working-class clients must help them work through unnecessary shame, developing the capacity to not experience shame for things that are not shameful, but are rather the result of oppression.

Thus, among the most interesting category for pastoral counselors is the capacity for persons who have been shamed by prevalent ideas about poor people, such as notions that the poor are a particular "type" of person, to not actually feel shame about their poverty. Such people understand the cultural and social factors of neoliberalism that have contributed to widespread poverty. Walker admits that this is a rare category—experiencing social shaming but feeling no shame—but I submit that it is an important category to foster through psychoeducation about the realities of poverty and through transforming the pastoral counselor's own perspective on poverty.

When Robert returned to Christina's office and saw the posters about economic inequity and the size of the new working class, he expressed appreciation for this information. Not that it was new information for him, but he had been bombarded with media images and political discourse about the laziness of the poor and their nature as cheaters from all sides. Even his previous employers seemed to treat him as less than human.

In this sense, understanding neoliberalism as a social-class project that has redistributed wealth to the upper five and one percent of the economy, and how this is a fairly recent change that began as a result of fiscal policies in the 1970s and 1980s, can help tremendously in reducing unnecessary shame that comes from being working class. Addressing the dynamics of shame means being willing to talk about the unnecessary shame of poverty, one of the more common experiences of working-class persons, and, besides an actual job, one of the important priorities they wish to address.

Managers and those in power frequently deploy shame to attempt to control the working class, and this is echoed by broad media approaches to represent the poor as deserving of their fate or asking for too much. For example, some managers use threats of removing certain goods, such as a break room, for minor violations, or punish an entire work crew for the mistake of one individual.[50] The active dynamics of shame mean that whenever a feeling is expressed, a person will be invalidated and be made to feel bad about having that feeling in the first place.

Working with the shame of social class in pastoral counseling means moving toward shame, accepting it as a reality, a nearly universal phenomenon that has purpose in certain contexts, but resisting its deployment for the purpose of social control. It also means noticing how shame is produced through the discourse of a particular context—its rules and regulations—and by what it says and leaves unsaid.

Robert described how one of his fellow workers in the factory was injured because Robert misplaced a tool. In this situation Robert felt appropriate guilt but his manager inculcated a sense of shame, calling him a "lousy worker" and stating, "I can't believe you did this. This is all your fault." Through discussing this encounter, Christina helped Robert resist the shame by exploring together the unfair conditions in the factory and how unpaid overtime had contributed to his stress.

Allowing the shame of social class to be voiced is a crucial dynamic that releases the energy of the shame-affect bind. When class is avoided as a topic of oppression or briefly mentioned, the powerful feelings associated with poverty, the dread of not being able to repay loans, the fear of having one's utilities turned off again, the anxiety about foreclosure, as well as the countless insults that come from being working class are subsumed into an experience of shame. The desire to avoid disgrace is the burying ground for emotions that have been tied to shame. There is a cost to hiding these feelings.

Discussing the power of social-class shame means naming what is difficult and uncovering it, thereby uncoupling the shame-affect bind and releasing energy for other experiences such as anger. Walker indicates that when poor persons could access anger they could organize to gain further rights, since they no longer blamed themselves for their experiences.[51] In engaging in these conversations, psychology that deals with interpersonal feelings is an important resource, even if it is inadequate to address the full conditions of working-class rights.

Robert stopped talking about himself as a failure in the sessions, and Christina noticed that there was more of a sparkle in his eye. Things continued to be hard as he looked for a job, but he seemed less likely to blame himself. "It's the system," he said. "It's not something wrong with me."

Psy-Complex Power in Pastoral Counseling Discourse

Pastoral counselors speak with clients but they also write about them, keeping notes about their problems and progress, tracking their medical and personal history, and documenting interactions about clients with other professionals. Counselors frequently engage in documentation about clients in files that they keep on them in locked cabinets, bringing them out only for consultation in case conference. Some theorists have argued, following Michel Foucault, that the practices of clinical file keeping and case conferences are themselves a form of social power.[52] Yet there are ways of working more transparently with clients that helps clients share power rather than simply having discourse used about them.

Christina met with her supervisor Frank about her clinical caseload and presented a short page about Robert and his progress. In it she offered the diagnosis "major depression" co-morbid with "substance abuse" and discussed how his economic situation was a risk factor for further relapses. In her discussion with her supervisor she shared some of the recent literature on how social suffering stemming from economic factors can contribute to mental and emotional distress. Her supervisor explained that he thought she was taking the client's side too much and that she needed to be more neutral. He wanted her to write a clinical note that de-emphasized the social factors and focused on Robert's mental illness. He also stressed that she needed to make a case for the medical necessity of his treatment in the event that the state decided to audit their practice. He made sure that a psychiatrist was prescribing Robert medication for his depression although Christina knew that he couldn't get the prescriptions filled because of a lack of finances.

The example noted previously shows the practice of management in a counseling center and exposes some of the ambiguities that have to do with the social context of the counseling center. In chapter 1, I described managers and professionals as being in a contradictory class location, with managers selling their authority for higher wages and professionals selling their skills and credentials for higher wages. In the example cited earlier, Christina has sold her professional skills and her manager has sold his authority. These professional classes have stresses of their own. There has even been research—described in chapter 1—that has shown that low-level managers have worse psychological health than their highly skilled employees, showing that the middle-of-the-class structure can be a difficult place to be in.

In the counseling context, social-class dynamics show up in the psychiatric discourse that is being used. Here we can see that Christina's work as a pastoral counselor puts her in the position of a psychological worker who must describe elements of Robert's story within a diagnostic frame and defend that frame so that care can be provided. By definition people who work in the psy-complex have an interest in defining people's problems as medical mental health problems so that they can treat them. As we saw in chapter 2, this diagnosis is a loose approximation of symptoms rather than direct access to the patient's experience.

Given what she knows about being in the working class and the psychic distress that stems from this, she is seeking ways to engage with Robert's suffering that will not simply manage symptoms, but address root causes, such as ongoing vulnerability to stress and trauma. Christina has been worrying about her class privilege since she began counseling Robert: if the working-class experience has to do with shame, contradictory class realities have to do with guilt. Just as it is unhelpful to silence shame, it is also unhelpful to silence guilt, since it usually speaks to a rupture in relationship that must be reconciled. An approach that emphasizes a client's psychological problems and adds social context as a footnote tends to veil the social- class dynamics of the counseling relationship itself.

As we saw earlier in the book, the psy-complex tends to use individualistic descriptions to explain people's mental problems and some of the most popular counseling treatments are highly individualistic. Once a person has begun treatment for depression, they are frequently measured with a set of scales such as the Beck Depression Inventory to measure progress during the treatment.

Such measures craft psychiatric disturbance into cognitive categories through a form of quantifiable measure. The author of the inventory Aaron Beck, the founder of Cognitive Behavioral Therapy (CBT), argued for the importance of internal evaluations, negative thought patterns tending to cast the world in all-or-nothing terms.[53] These all-or-nothing terms are described as negative thoughts or distorted cognitions that can then be rendered transparent to both the counselor and the client through a discussion of the client's flawed thinking. The therapist then works to progressively making the person's worldview more rational. Becoming healthier is thus described as becoming more independent, autonomous, and in control of one's thought processes.

CBT attempts to render the thought processes of the client visible to the counselor by projects such as homework in which a person evaluates their mistaken thoughts and explores how they have exaggerated their problems.[54] Most counseling treatment nowadays, including the depression scale mentioned earlier, are based upon some variation of this approach. Widely evaluated as a successful evidence-based therapy, CBT focuses on the thoughts and rationalization of an individual sufferer and allows it to be coded.

The process of CBT places the counselor in the position of rational agent over the disordered, flawed, and irrational thinking of the client. Rather than the client's thoughts being construed as an understandable response to an impossible situation of chronic sorrow, pervasive disempowerment, and systemic injustice, flawed ideas are posited that exist in the client's mind and create dysfunctional forms of behavior. Counseling requires a kind of Stoic therapy on the self, in which one's feelings and desires are processed rationally, while all along the social suffering that contributed to distress is implicitly minimized by the process. For example, perhaps people are afraid because there is something to be afraid of, rather than because of irrational thinking.

CBT has become popular in managed care in the United States because it offers quantifiable approach to account for some severe and intractable mental difficulties. As one social worker maintained, his supervisor coached him to use CBT skills with a family that had fought over a loaf of bread.[55] Deconstructing irrational beliefs is not important when the cupboard is bare.

What if a client's negative beliefs are not irrational but a result of the profound mistreatment that stems from social-class oppression? Chronic trauma and stress of this kind cannot simply be wished away by more positive thinking or by reframing a client's difficulties as irrational. It is quite instructive to note what CBT does not measure. It does not measure the conditions in which people work or aspects of stress in their daily schedule such as a lengthy or unpredictable commute on public transportation. It does not measure the impact of microaggressions or structural disempowerment. The central presumption is that, whatever social and structural factors may have contributed to the form of mental distress which persons' face, the primary problem now is that it has distorted the thinking in their heads.

Building from this approach, the inner world is then brought out for another to see and judge. Because of the pervasive and ongoing nature of social class, significant oppressive factors such as economics are minimized in CBT: what is emphasized is the internal thought process that follows from experiences of oppression. CBT is described here as simply one example of a range of interventions that tend to treat the minds of individuals—such interventions are necessarily the bread-and-butter of counseling. The popularity of CBT, and its widely held acceptance as an evidence-based therapy, is rooted in the efficiency-based schema of managed care.

Some pastoral counselors work in situations closely allied to the *psy-complex,* but even these spaces can be sites of resistance. In his article "Surveillance and Government of the Welfare Recipient," Ken Moffatt notes how social workers in an office in a North American city investigated the people who came to see them to determine whether or not their clients were eligible for welfare. He notes how these social workers would sometimes resist the system by refusing to listen to a client who was disclosing earning a little extra money from a family member or by working. Moffatt notes these practices as addressing social control. Although it is important not to go as far as sanctioning illegality, it is also significant to find ways of working that resist the limits of the psy-complex.

In this section I have described how counselors engage in the *psy-complex* when they render the social suffering of clients into an exclusively individualistic frame. They may be most likely to do so when they become anxious about the client's progress. I have argued that therapeutic interventions such as file keeping, diagnostic language, and case conferences about clients without them being present, have the effect of further individualizing and disempowering clients. By contrast, there are ways in which counselors can advocate for clients in the social sphere and connect them to group resources to challenge their experience of working-class oppression.

Advocacy and Group Work as a Stance for Working-Class Counseling

Thus far in the chapter we have focused on the interpretive role that counselors play, but here we should offer that pastoral counselors could also become advocates for their clients. Helpful aspects of this interpretive, question-asking approach can be combined with approaches that more directly address the context of being in the working and contingent classes. Some important voices in the pastoral counseling field have critiqued the idea that counselors can act as simply a "neutral" reflecting partner. Rather, even supposedly impartial conversations are implicated in social and cultural dynamics. For example, Watkins Ali has suggested that counselors must also play the role of advocate sometimes.[56]

There have been several recent counseling approaches that combine advocacy for working-class persons with counseling approaches drawn from the psychological sciences. For example, Ramón Rojano's Community Family Therapy (CFT) approach puts getting out of poverty as a primary goal of the therapy process and encourages clients who have done so to exert leadership in their communities. The first goal of CFT is "moving family income above the poverty line" and thus "to move people from poverty to middle class."[57] Therapy proceeds in three levels, the first of which engages personal issues such as self-esteem, the second of which equips clients with a community of resources and religious supports, and the third of which asks the client to give back to the community. For example, one woman whose husband had left her and was living below the poverty line was eventually able to volunteer at her child's school, which itself led to a job offer.[58]

Doing this kind of counseling requires a perceptual shift away from expert-guidance to accompaniment. In CFT the therapists have to see the client as a peer "deserving the same rights and opportunities as themselves" and also have "a personal connection with providers of at least ten different services."[59] He maintains that therapists may have to work in spaces outside counseling such as schools, homes, or other public venues. The first stated priority for a CFT therapist is the relief of poverty. The community resources that the therapist engages with help with this goal. Although CFT addresses the suffering of working and contingent-class clients by attempting to bring them out of poverty, it does not explicitly examine the conditions of work or the dynamics of social class in the therapy. Nevertheless, CFT is one of the first counseling methods to place explicit emphasis on the relief of poverty as a therapeutic goal.

Likewise, a therapeutic community of working and contingent-class women who have faced depression, Reaching Out About Depression (ROAD) have explicitly addressed the intersection between mental health and poverty in their communities. Undergirded by feminist ethics, they note that the experience of poverty has disproportionately affected women both through stress and trauma.[60] The gathering began as the result of Kitchen Table Project, which were conversations among low-income women about the needs of their communities. The city of Cambridge began sponsoring weekly dinners—with childcare provided—where women could talk about the micro- and macro-elements of their lives.[61]

All members of the collective work together to facilitate each meeting and the goal of the meeting is "collective empowerment" and "participatory action."[62] At the end of a series of meetings the group has a voice and engages in community action. These actions can be as varied as creating a cookbook for how to eat well with little money or inviting community leaders to hear their concerns.

This group is led by c/s/x activists who engage in community action and intervention to change the conditions of class oppression in their community. It is worth noting that this group is also engaging in intersectional gender analysis through its use of feminist themes. The group has bypassed psychiatric models of depression to focus on a biopsychosocial model that explicitly addresses poverty. Although it has been a powerful assistance to many, ROAD is dependent on outside funding and thus requires continued institutional support.

In approaches like these, the individual client's psychology is only one part of a larger picture, which includes cultural factors and clients are empowered to directly address the conditions that contribute to their suffering. Such approaches highlight collaboration between client and therapist rather than treating each client as an individual with a psychopathology. A shortcoming of these approaches is that they do not go far enough in addressing the core conditions of capitalism, since rather than simply offering "uplift" into an existing system, we also need to advocate to change the system itself. Working-class persons who are seeking voice and power in their lives are best helped by approaches to therapy that include advocacy and empowerment specifically pertaining to social class.

It is important to foster transparency to increase the power held by working-class clients. As I analyzed in the previous section, in much counseling practice, counselors do not work alone but operate in close cooperation with the state, the juvenile court system, the penal system, the welfare system, and other social service agencies. Naming this interdependence of institutions is one way of acknowledging that pastoral counseling uses power in its very practices. The language about the client circulates among these various agencies rather than remaining in the client's file. Rendering this process of language-distribution more evident means sharing with clients about who is involved in their process of clinical management and giving them access to the conversations about their treatment—even where this treatment is mandated—so that more ethical counseling practices can result.[63]

There are also ways of working in groups that can challenge the lack of transparency. In Sweden, a team working on the problem of sexual abuse of children in a poor rural community began to meet with all the stakeholders in a process called a "reflecting team" where all the members of a team are available for discourse about a client. A reflecting team is a process in which various stakeholders are gathered and take turns listening to each other, in the "reflective position."[64] When they respond to what they heard, they avoid clinical judgments, name-calling, or pathologizing, but make their remarks in the first person using comments such as "it seems to me."[65] They describe a process of intentional reflection that is quite different from how power is typically used in sexual abuse allegation cases in the United States.

> During that first meeting one of us interviews the different people present. Other team members are in the room in a reflective position. When we have discussed the premise for our meeting we make sure to ask those most uncomfortable or afraid how they will feel safe to express themselves... First we talk with the social worker, because he/she as referring agent... owns the problem... we then try to find out whether the different family members in any way agree with the social worker and in what ways they don't agree... We then ask the social workers to be specific as to what will happen if the family chooses not to cooperate... we stipulate that we will not discuss the case with the referring person unless the parents are informed or present.[66]

They describe the consequences of working in this way in a particular situation of intimate partner violence. When the social agency asked the wife and children's therapist if the previously violent father could be back in touch with his children, the counselors mediated the claims of the father via the social service agency. They did this by using videotaped sessions of the father. The spouse and children would watch the father talk on videotape. Then they videotaped the spouse and children talking and shared it with the father. In the videotapes, the children and the father each got a chance to state their fears and desires. At the end of a three-year process, the father has been in a room with the therapists and their children two times and find that "they have a lot to talk about." "Nowadays they are satisfied with about four meetings a year."[67]

In another situation counselors, social workers, foster parents, biological parents, and children all met together to discuss the possibility of a biological mother being reunited with her children. In this meeting the children described what "safety" would feel like for them. Social workers defined what would work legally for the mother to care for her children and the children got to voice their concerns. Although the mother eventually returned to drinking, children were able to offer their voices so that legal authorities that held the power over their destinies could hear them. For example, one of the children said, "I don't want to be used by the social agency to determine whether my mother is healthy or not" and another made a practical suggestion, "Can my mother get a telephone from the social agency so that I can phone her easily?"[68] One of the social workers expressed appreciation for the meetings because "I have an impossible job acting both as the police...and at the same time helping you and your children."[69]

The Swedish therapeutic team described their unorthodox method—building bridges across social service agencies rather than simply allowing each member of the legal, psychiatric, and social worker community exert their own form of control. They also showed how this model of working came from the contingencies of their practical situation in a rural community. "Because we lived and worked in the health care system of a small community, we shared the collective beliefs and 'knew' the histories and fates of many families for generations" and this meant that there were multiple encounters with families in the community besides those in just the professional setting, a situation that led these counselors to find more collaborative ways of working.[70]

Sharing information in this way shortcuts the suspicion about public services. This approach often leads to empowerment since it "liberates parents to find new ways to act even during difficult life crises, including societal control."[71] As such, because families—even presumably dangerous parents and children—are able to sit in a room together and talk with the various stakeholders in their lives, such as relatives, teachers, friends, lawyers, and social workers, there is a situation in which persons are less likely to find themselves the object of power and more likely to come to collaborative forms of working that honor the resources and responsibilities of various parties. Reflecting team models offer a way of speaking across community agencies about the problems in people's lives. There are also some approaches that have begun to empower people to address the core conditions that contribute to their suffering—economic injustice. Some approaches to counseling in the United States have begun to explicitly address social class.

Pastoral counselors who are already overwhelmed by the work that they are doing in their institutions, dealing with the pressures of documentation and case management, may wonder about the feasibility about adding advocacy to their already overwhelmed schedules. Nevertheless, part of the stress of pastoral counseling comes from working to address the pain of social circumstances which will continue, and pastoral counselors can avoid burnout by working simultaneously to address the social suffering that persons are facing and change the conditions that contribute to that suffering. Additionally, the models provided earlier also empower the client and thus lead to less of an exclusive sense of therapist responsibility for a client.

For example, Christina began to be involved in both a local interfaith organization and a Jobs for Justice group in her area. As the result of their labor activism, this community organization got a major employer to raise their compensation by two dollars an hour. When Robert was hired by the organization a month later, he had more of a cushion to support himself, leading him to reach out to his children again.

In cases in which counselees see their primary problems to be psychiatric concerns, such as mental illness or addiction, a counselor can still work as an advocate for that client by getting them the support that they need while also organizing to change the conditions in which these forms of suffering were exacerbated. Even as the counselor seeks to give the client psychological help, they need to challenge the limiting metaphors and narratives of biomedical psychiatry. The most helpful thing for the client will likely be supportive relationships that mirror social reality back to the client.

By working to address the conditions of labor and challenge capitalism, the pastoral counselor also creates a stronger social safety net for future clients. At times there is a risk that a counselor may begin interpreting the social context of suffering in terms that do not match with the client's understanding. At times, simply naming the extent of suffering: "I've noticed that a lot of my clients are struggling to make ends meet and get really stressed out about it," can broaden the context and help clients feel as if they are not alone.

In this section we have seen how pastoral counselors can directly address issues such as poverty, and how they can help clients work together as groups who are interested in addressing the intersection of mental illness and economic realities, and how they can work collaboratively in reflecting teams to share power and build voice. If clients are not bothered by psychological problems alone but by a host of community concerns that interfere with their well-being, a counselor may feel comfortable showing up at a labor meeting, a protest, or a school board meeting in the role of a concerned community member seeking to foster the client's mental health. Likewise, they may begin writing letters about the community concerns facing their constituents and clients to representatives in government, since their professional status lends them credence.

If pastoral counselors are indeed in a *contradictory class position,* sharing elements of both the working and owning class, they can use some of these contradictions to the client's advantage rather than being paralyzed by them. Rieger has noted that there is often a subtle equating of social power with theological power, but that we need to challenge this tendency.[72] By using their power as professionals to address the class needs of clients, pastoral counselors will be moving closer to solidarity with their working-class clients. This echoes some significant themes from the early pastoral counseling movement, the traditions of the transformation of the social order with the concerns of justice.

Recovering Social Teaching for Pastoral Counseling

In the early twentieth century, Protestant ministers who labored in working-class communities sought religious solutions to the ills associated with poverty and proposed a Social Gospel. This approach to Christianity argued that the Kingdom of God was not merely something reserved for final days, but that transformations in human justice could be part of God's plan in the present. For early figures such as Washington Gladden and Walter Rauschenbusch, salvation was not limited to an individual's faith but had to include redemption from current material conditions such as poverty, child labor, and homelessness. As such, theology could not be separated from the social condition of persons' lives.

The time is right for reclamation of the social gospel as an influence on pastoral care and counseling. The earliest counseling clinics in urban areas meant to address psychological and spiritual concerns in people's lives.

The conditions in modern society mirror early twentieth-century inequity. Pamela Couture notes how income inequity is similar today to the levels where it was when the Social Gospel became popular. She argues that women and children and minorities are often poorer in the United States and maintains that "at the heart of these issues is the suffering of individuals and families and therefore, issues of pastoral care are directly embedded in these conditions."[73] Addressing this poverty cannot be an addendum to pastoral care and counseling but must form the heart of our approach to it.

Even before the Social Gospel movement was taking place in Protestantism, Pope Leo XIII issued a statement *Rerum novarum* that protested the conditions of industrial workers. This began a centuries-long engagement by the Catholic Church in economic matters, culminating in Pope Francis' emphasis on critiquing global injustice stemming from runaway capitalism.[74] Among the strongest contribution of this tradition has been ethical and theological reflection on "property rights, human rights, solidarity, subsidiarity, and participation."[75] Arguing that labor had value and should be honored apart from exploitation in an instrumental sense, it gave a language for valuing the distinctive contribution that workers make. This tradition lifts up ethical ideals such as the *common good* in complex relationship with the individual's self-interest. Catholic ethicists such as John A. Ryan were among the first to advocate for the living wage.[76]

Although there are some problems with these traditions—for example the Social Gospel movement offered a vision of White Protestant salvation as part of social transformation and the Catholic Social Teaching tradition essentialized and thus stereotyped women[77]—these held in common a vision of how the economic conditions of society were fundamentally theological. This was because economics could not be separated from the human person in relationship with God and with others.

Understanding the importance of economics does not place everything on the immanent plane or even suggest that one has to choose between transcendence and immanence. As Joerg Rieger states, *"transcendence* has to do not with otherworldliness but with transcending a particular form of immanence that is determined by the status quo (e.g., the Roman Empire, establishment religion) in order to embrace a different form of immanence (on a stable, on the margins, with the 'least of these')."[78] The shared commitments of these traditions argue that religion is something that should change social life in the here-and-now.

Many persons of faith are inspired by theological arguments that highlight fundamental aspects of what it means to be a person, such as "the inviolable dignity of every human person... the essential centrality of community, and the significance of human action."[79] Addressing economic realities is crucial to allowing this dignity-through-relationship to come to the fore.

It is important to return to some fundamental anthropological principles such as the notion of solidarity, participation, and social sin, in order to reclaim a theological vantage point for addressing social class within pastoral counseling. If persons are not monads, and if their mental and spiritual well-being cannot be conceptualized in a vacuum apart from other persons, then there are theological principles that undergird how a pastoral counselor approaches their work with clients. This does not mean that clients need to share their counselor's faith in order for the counseling to be effective. Rather, a theological lens that foregrounds human dignity and attends to the common good gives one of the most promising frameworks for addressing the social/spiritual needs of people in the twenty-first century, inspiring and undergirding ethical action.[80]

Robert in his fourth session described how he had lost faith after praying to God for work and not finding any. His faith used to be an important part of his life when he had his family and factory job, but it started to make less and less sense to him as he had hit the "hard times." He still prays sometimes and sees Jesus as having more in common with him that with rich folks. She has a feeling he is looking for faith. Spirituality as it is commonly conceived in the twenty-first century makes little sense to him.

Christina began to realize how class oppression could contribute to a crisis of faith, and she considered how it was bound up with the notion of shame. The more Robert blamed himself for his economic failings, the further he felt from God. Christina began to realize that addressing social-class shame was part and parcel of addressing Robert's faith, which makes sense when we consider that embracing shame is a significant aspect of the spiritual journey. As Donald Capps argues in a discussion about shame in the Christian life, "to put our shameful selves aside is to dissociate ourselves experientially from the shame of the cross. On the other hand, to embrace our shameful self is to identify with Jesus and thereby experience God as no longer hidden."[81] Addressing shame directly means identifying with Jesus who was a marginalized working-class person, always at risk of being shamed by able to resist this shame.

Christina found that it was only through addressing social-class shame that she could communicate hope—what she considered as fundamental to her religious orientation—in situations where hopelessness was pervasive.

Within this framework, she began orienting her counseling to the *common good* and not merely to the individual suffering. For this reason Christina joined workers rights efforts in her community, since she saw that the issues of ethical or religious development that she hoped to see in her client's lives could only be achieved with persistent social activism for the rights and well-being of workers. As Dorothy Day once wrote, echoing the sentiments of Catholic Worker founder Peter Maurin, the efforts of the Worker were meant "to build that society where it is easier for people to be good."[82]

The two parts of Christina's approach to counseling—fostering human dignity and a sense of purpose or vocation—were each funded by her theological commitments. She believed that Robert's dignity and purpose were part of who God had created Robert to be. Yet helping that purpose be lived out required challenging the social systems that made him feel, in words drawn from Bauman in chapter 1, increasingly "redundant" in the new economy. Directly grappling with social suffering brought faith to life. Her principles continued to draw her to working-class activism to alleviate the suffering that brought Robert to counseling in the first place. This meant doing preventative pastoral counseling—making it more likely that people would have what they need, making it less likely that they would suffer.

The underlying principle behind her approach to counseling was that God loves each person and wants them to feel loved, but for persons who have been profoundly oppressed by their working-class position, they can struggle to perceive this reality and even the sentiment can ring as inauthentic. As Gustavo Gutiérrez, founder of liberation theology stated, the central question of his life's work has been how you could authentically say to the poor that God loved them.[83] It is only possible to lay the groundwork for the conditions of God's love by creating practical moments in which people's needs can be met and so they can have the opportunity to fully experience God's presence and care.

Structural sin and salvation are thus intimately bound up with the practice of pastoral counseling. Recovering the Social Gospel roots of the discipline allows for important connections to social circumstances to come to the fore. It raises the issue of changing the circumstances of social harm so that persons are more able to live out their dignity and purpose. It also increases the reliability and authenticity of one's religious commitments to those who come for counseling. Removing barriers and obstacles to daily survival also makes it more likely that people will have an opportunity to flourish in their psychic lives and contribute to their communities. Ideally, it is not the church as an outside entity advocating the rights of the working class, but it is people in their own class positions raising their voice and advocating for their rights.

In order to do this, it is helpful to remember that the founding members of the Social Gospel movement argued that we must simultaneously address social sin in order to foster psychological maturity and religious redemption so that society could be changed to more rightly reflect God's purposes. In pastoral counseling, this means addressing the social circumstances such as economic inequity, a lack of access to social goods such as education and counseling, and fostering opportunities for all persons to engage with the traditions of their religious faiths.

Conclusion

In this chapter we have seen how pastoral counseling, a practice of counseling developed in 1963 under the auspices of the Association of Pastoral Counseling, can be a site from which to develop solidarity and working-class alliances by addressing the cross-class relationship that occurs in counseling.

Pastoral counseling is the kind of relationship that is established through a client's invitation to a therapist to help them interpret their lives, and I have maintained that it should increasingly include elements of advocacy in addition to psychological care. I have argued for the necessity of addressing class in counseling. At times this can mean knowing about resources for low-rent housing or transportation. At other times this can mean helping persons to address the unnecessary shame that comes from poverty.

Counselors are often called upon to make individualistic attributions of identity to their clients, such as giving them a mental health diagnosis. In these circumstances, a client can be individualized by being written about in a file, having case conferences "done" on them, and increasingly come to be seen as the problem. This approach, an effect of working in the *psy-complex,* can be exacerbated if the counselor is responsible for determining a client's eligibility for benefits.

I have argued that naming social class in counseling is possible in ways that transcend the *psy-complex* and instead begin to speak of the embodied experience of being in a particular social class. For example, questions that help describe the relational nature of class begin to indicate that social class is a series of relationships: owners would not be able to operate corporations without the cooperation of workers in positions of subjugation.

Such a public psychology should be used to help working-class people resist unnecessary shame of poverty despite being actively shamed. Using elements of education and support and discussing the ubiquity of poverty, counselors can help deconstruct popularly held notions about persons in the working class. This means challenging how frequently shame is bound to other emotions, allowing feelings like anger to be released for the sake of social activism. What is often at stake is not merely psychological health but one's spiritual life, as one comes to be able to identify with a working-class Christ and thus reduce the shame and stigma of poverty.

Pastoral counseling can include social change to address poverty as a first-order priority by making rising above the poverty line a therapeutic goal and by fostering conversations in groups about the relationship between social class and mental distress. In this sense, a counselor is a facilitator, advocate, and fellow citizen who helps empower the clients to change the conditions in which social oppression happens.

Christina's pastoral counseling with Robert, like so many counseling encounters, did not end with a smooth resolution. After losing a low-wage service job he dropped out of the counseling and she did not have a chance to see him again for therapy. Nevertheless, Christina's orientation to her work profoundly changed. She no longer tried to confront the negative thoughts of clients through an individualistic cognitive model, but sought to actively change the conditions that lead to their suffering. She began studying the link between poverty and mental distress, a connection that was not emphasized in her education. She helped discuss and deconstruct their shame, talking actively about the conditions of class struggle in our society. The surroundings of her office, the paintings and posters on the wall, displayed that she was committed not only to psychological health but also working rights, a key condition to psychological well-being for so many in our society.

CHAPTER 5

The Counter-Conducts of Pastoral Power

A pastor welcomes a family into her study, stating that she will be able to meet with them for one or two sessions before she refers them to another counselor. They describe the struggles of being "down in the dumps" ever since the wife was fired from her work unceremoniously. Just at the same time, this family faced their rents skyrocketing. The minister thinks they came in for counseling because she had begun to share economy stories from the pulpit, discussing the effect of the downturn on everyone.

This pastor initially brainstormed getting a local charity to help with this family's rent, but heard later that week from a dozen other families whose rents were going up. Although the minister had initially approached this as a family counseling issue and had been planning to refer to a couple's counselor, she began to think that practical financial considerations needed to come first. When the minister began that conversation, it lead to the community organizing efforts to foster affordable housing in their city. Because of the intense public pressure, the landlords relented two months later. With the housing situation sorted out, they went to see the pastor for a follow up: "There's less stress in our lives now," they said. "We also have more purpose in our relationship since we have both gotten involved in faith-based advocacy."

In previous chapters we have explored the extent of mental distress in our times, the limitations of an exclusively biomedical approach to treating it, testimony from mental patients about their experiences of survivorship, as well as pastoral counseling as a way of resisting exclusively medical models of psychiatry and fostering solidarity.

In this chapter we offer a fresh vision for how ministry can be a site of constructive power using the philosophy of Michel Foucault, especially his notion of the counter-conducts of pastoral power: *mysticism, community, asceticism, Scripture,* and *eschatology*.[1] The distinctive contribution of this chapter is to show how elements that have traditionally been considered to fall in the realm of spirituality are actually at the heart of pastoral care. Foucault noted that these elements were "border practices" within Christianity that allowed for a challenge to the unjust imposition of power. Pastoral care in neoliberal times requires an integrative approach that addresses both spirituality and oppression together, and Foucault's notion of the counter-conducts of pastoral power provides a well-suited conceptual tool for the task.

Some may be surprised to find such traditionally Christian themes in the work of a critical theorist such as Foucault. Yet, his central concerns were shaped by his religious heritage. "When someone commented that Foucault sounded 'very Christian' he replied, 'Yes, I have a very strong Christian, Catholic background, and I am not ashamed.'"[2] In his discussion of the ways in which we are shaped as subjects and how we come to see our identities formed, his Christian heritage was an important influence on his intellectual development. He once cited Marx, whose oft-cited epigram "religion is the opiate of the people" actually leaves out the full meaning when he described religion as "the spirit of a world without a spirit."[3]

People may be familiar with a more negative reading of Foucault. In this understanding, Foucault's emphasis on power provides a helpful lens for how we ought to interpret the repressive use of power, even power that seems to lead to liberation. He maintains that even as we attempt to craft a more just and equitable world, we may be fixing people through discourse—often the labels that we use for persons only explain a small part of their experience and can be constrictive.

He saw that pastoral ministry could be the site of such a shaping of subjectivity and argued that there have always been "border practices" in Christianity that challenge these forms of social control. Power is not extrinsic to theology but coterminous with it. In this chapter we explore Foucault's hopeful notion of a power found within practices of Christian communities that could be used to transform subjectivity.

My argument is that we must utilize these border practices to open up the reflective space of our religious communities to more broadly challenge neoliberal capitalism and the impoverishment and indignities of social class. While Foucault may not have imagined the counter-conducts of pastoral power being put to use to analyze the suffering stemming from economic oppression, neither would he have predicted the shape of neoliberalism on the global stage. Yet his notions provide transformative potential for these times. His approach actually is well suited to times of depersonalization and desperation since they highlight both the importance of relationships of love between God and the Christian community.

Foucault noted the structure of pastoral power, how it relied upon models of shepherding a whole community that required a minister to take responsibility for the entire community as well as the individual. Suspicious of the religious authority inherent in this responsibility, he points to strategies for resisting it. In our work, we can exercise pastoral power more responsibility if we address Foucault's suspicions. Likewise, we can utilize his counter-conducts of pastoral power as one of the most helpful means of restoring liberative power to communities of faith.

My thesis in this chapter is that pastoral ministry is a central site from which advocacy for the whole community can be engaged, and, in doing so, ministers can transform that conditions that have contributed to persons' psychic suffering. This transformation is at the heart of pastoral power. Helping persons name and resist the suffering that comes from living in a neoliberal era, ministers can learn to use elements of counter-conduct to help communities thrive. Communities of faith, rather than ministers themselves, are the key actors in pastoral power. When readers are finished with this chapter they will be prepared to foster such resistance in their own communities.

Ministers Monitoring Mental Illness

There is greater awareness of the problem of mental illness among ministers today; including teaching clergy the signs of emotional suffering that they see everyday.[4] Evangelical churches are beginning to discuss mental illness within a biomedical framework.[5] These trends exemplify that ministers are important interpreters of social suffering in their communities, yet there is scant attention to the impact of the economic conditions of social class in this time of mental suffering.

Rick Warren's Saddleback Church recently hosted a conference entitled "Mental Health and the Church" in which psychiatrists and ministers gathered to destigmatize mental illness.[6] Warren's son's tragic suicide was the impetus for the conference. In the conference, participants argued that mental health care from a biomedical point of view was compatible with Christian approaches to healing. As one presenter argued, God has placed the tools of science at our disposal. Testimonies from consumers of mental health care featured "manly" and "womanly" stories of reaching out and asking for help as a sign of strength and compassion. Warren argued that churches could become places for healing if pastors would reach out to other experts who could provide psychological counseling and psychotropic drugs. Co-funded by NAMI, this conference highlighted a biological view of mental illness rather than emphasizing social or psychological factors.

Warren notes that the church is often the first place people go to when they are in distress. Rather than approaching a medical professional, they turn to clergy, since the church is a place of hope. As he says in his typical catch-phrase fashion, "We're hope dispensers."[7] In order for the church to truly function as a hopeful place it must grapple with the concrete realities that people face rather than glossing over them.

Warren notes that there are social factors that enter into the picture—"The economy doesn't work perfectly."[8] Yet he states that this is because "everything in the world is broken by sin."[9] This blame-everyone strategy does not discuss the specific role the economy might play in the rates of mental distress or how ministry could be geared to directly address these stressors. Rather than triaging the symptoms of mental distress, the church could be a place where the actual causes of mental illness could be addressed. The harm that the economy can cause in the mental distress people face is thus generalized, discussed in terms of universal sin rather than specific harms that have been committed.

The implication of Warren's conference is that we know what mental illness is and how to treat it, so the key thing to do is simply reduce stigma and increase access. From this point of view, it is a disease of the brain and genes that affects our communities. Helping people who suffer from an individual ailment is goal, but presumably this is something the church can easily take up if the government is not helping.

Saddleback's mission meets an important need since it helps clergypersons know about the extent of emotional distress. According to the National Comorbidity Survey, ministers are contacted for mental health care a quarter of the time, while psychiatrists only 16 percent of the time, and a quarter of these are said to have serious mental illness.[10] In the African American community, women are more likely than men to seek out clergy, while they are far less likely to discuss economic problems as part of that consultation.[11] Clergy report that they spend between 10 and 20 percent of their work doing counseling, about eight hours a week.[12]

It seems that Warren and his NAMI-funded conference are correct that ministers have a distinctive role to play in their communities, and the fact that the troubled seek clergy more than psychiatrists gives them a kind of power. But this power itself might have some problematic aspects. At times, ministers who treat persons with mental illness might come to see them as an identity—*a sick individual*—and thus miss the broader cultural surroundings, which through factors such as economic oppression, contributes significantly to the cause and the course of emotional distress. In what follows, we describe how ministers come to have the power to manage a territory and how this power connects with the kinds of interpretations that ministers make in pastoral care. Foucault cannily understood the kind of power that minister's have and proposed a model for understanding it. I add to his model a three-part definition of pastoral power and discuss the impact of ministerial discourse.

Pastoral Power

In the middle period of his life, during the interval between the publication of the first volume of *The History of Sexuality* and the second, Foucault lectured extensively on governmental power and studied the conceptual reach of the state through practices of measurement. The logic of the discourse of health was fostered through the study of large populations who for the first time could be measured on graphs of health and normality. He offered concepts like "governmentality" and "biopower" which have increasingly been taken up by scholars in a variety of fields.[13] Foucault was not so much critical of pastoral power as he was of its use by the state. He was interested in how the modern forms of state government echoed and built upon earlier religious themes.

Pastoral power means the capacity to govern people as a whole and as individuals that is seen in the ancient metaphor for shepherding. "The pastoral relationship in its full and positive form is therefore essentially the relationship of God to man [sic]."[14] Rather than being defined by its might, pastoral power is characterized by duty and humble beneficence, and is marked by a willingness to sacrifice for the flock. This notion of sacrifice heightens the minister's power over the flock. Being a minister requires a double focus, thus "keep[ing] [one's] eye on all and on each, *Omnes et Singulatum*" is one of the most significant aspects of ministry.[15]

One of the characteristics of this relationship is that the flock is symbolized as *on the move,* a fact that Foucault illustrates with an anecdote. Citing Plato's figure of the *Statesman,* he suggests that Moses was chosen to shepherd the people out of Egypt "because he knew how to graze his sheep."[16] For this reason he knew how to guide his people.

This reference to transition means that pastors have a unique role that is only heightened in times of transition.

Traditionally the discipline of pastoral counseling has fostered what have been seen as shepherding activities: "healing, guiding, sustaining, and reconciling."[17] These activities are supposed to have been undertaken with "an attitude of tender and solicitous concern" by the minister, who, by virtue of the symbolic power vested in them, is frequently seen as a representative of God.[18] Yet Foucault reminds us that each activity of care, especially when accompanied by the sanction of religious respectability, can also be a form of control. He says it tersely, "Pastoral power is a power of care."[19]

The object of pastoral power in Foucault's understanding is to hold together the salvation of the flock as a whole with the care of each individual sheep—the principle of *Omnes et Singulatum*, or "of all and of each." He quotes early Christian authors, from Ambrose to John of Chrysostom, to show how this responsibility for the salvation of the souls is likened to an "economy of souls."[20] Feeding, guarding, guiding, and becoming responsible for the community is the heart of pastoral power, which for Foucault is an individualizing power. The test of pastoral power is whether the clergy will leave the whole to care for one single sheep (Lk. 15:4).

While there is more that could be said about this depiction, it is an essentially helpful image of the link between ministerial authority and responsibility. In ethical discussions, it is commonly held that pastoral ministry must include a responsibility to safeguard the trust and intimacy of the congregants. While some ministers try to downplay their power by acting just like their congregants, this actually promotes pastoral power. It does this because ministers have heightened access to their congregations.[21]

One of Foucault's chief concerns about pastoral power is that it is too individualizing. Ministers hear the shame, anxiety, and depression of congregants and may treat them as troubled persons. Yet when clergy are called upon to respond to these feelings, they also envision them as what Anne Cvetkovich calls "public feelings," presumably intrapsychic realities that are inextricably bound up with the signs of our times.[22] This means holding together the broader community analysis even as they engage in one-on-one care. In order to understand counselees' feelings, ministers must help their congregants achieve outsight as much as insight.[23]

Ministers have symbolic authority in their communities that comes with certain privileges. By educating the clergy in an exclusively medical model of mental illness and then expecting them to refer to psychiatrists in their community, Warren capitalizes on this symbolic authority, the capacity to shepherd a flock in a territory. While ministerial authority seems to have declined somewhat in recent years, it is still a reality in many parts of the country. Ministers utilize language, in conversation with mental emotionally distressed people, that help shape what it means for them to be a person. This tremendous power is what Foucault points to when he notes how "ministry" ambiguously refers to both pastoral leadership and a government post: shepherding people in a spiritual sense is not so different from governing them in a secular one.[24]

A chief objection to this image of pastoral power is that Foucault has misrepresented many of the feelings and intentions of ministers by depicting clergy as having control over the souls of their flock. Clergy often sacrifice greatly for their calling and it seems paradoxical to suggest that they have a kind of power that comes from this sacrifice. Foucault suggests that pastoral power ironically is what arises from the joint phenomena of sacrifice and responsibility. Derived from the accompaniment of the flock through dangerous and difficult times ministers get power through the renunciation of power. I am convinced that this power is not merely negative or controlling, but can be used to effectively guide the community to its own best empowerment.

It is already clear that I am taking images from Foucault's discussion of pastoral power and putting them to my own use. In my analysis here pastoral power can certainly be misused but it can also be a legitimate authority, earned through established trust across time, in which people help their community be fed and grow closer to God and to their neighbors. I lift up the image of sustenance and argue that ministry must combine the approach to helping congregants find material sustenance as well as spiritual food.[25] Foucault was concerned about government usurping the power of the pastorate and my purpose with this analysis is more limited: to explore the textures of pastoral power and how it might be effectively used to accompany and guide a community.

Let me give a brief example of someone using pastoral power effectively to shepherd a flock. In rural New York, Presbyterian minister Janet Adair Hanson organized an interdenominational congregation-based community organization (CBCO) to address poverty. She interviewed more than 250 people in the community, asking about their most pressing needs, which turned out to be health care for young people. Hanson literally ministered to the flock by going from house to house with her organizing group and asking people concrete questions about the material conditions of their lives. We can see Foucault's principles of

Omnes et Signulatum at work here. In providing care for the whole community she cared for each individual member. Likewise, when she saw individual members in counseling she thought about the whole community as she heard their stories. Hanson's pastoral power consisted of her religious authority, which she used in managing a territory, but also her legitimacy from travelling with persons in her community for a period of time, seeking to feed and sustain them in both material and spiritual ways. In an important fashion, her religious authority contributed to her ability to organize this group to meet concrete needs in their communities.

Three Sources of Pastoral Power

In this section I go beyond Foucault's analysis to propose three sources of pastoral power. The extent of pastoral power is shaped by three interlocking sources that I submit are crucial to understanding the interpretive framework of pastoral power. While Foucault primarily emphasized symbolic religious authority, there are also two other factors that contribute to pastoral power. I maintain that these sources of pastoral power are the trust that derives from travelling with people over a period of time, symbolic authority, and shared cultural location.

First, since pastoral power concerns the transitional nature of God's people as a flock, the power is impacted by how much time a leader has travelled with people. One clergy person who sought to make her congregation more inclusive of persons with nontraditional sexualities during her first year with them was unsuccessful. Yet after three years she was able to make this change. This is the temporal dimension of ministry. For people suffering from mental distress because of the new economy, they may not trust their minister in the first several years to talk about taboo subjects like finances. Yet after a period of time, they may begin to share their worries about foreclosure and having the utilities shut off. This does not mean that chaplains who minister in episodic ways do not have pastoral power, but that either their power is drawn primarily from the other two sources or they have remained in the same community for so long they become a trusted figure.

Second, the extent of pastoral power is also impacted by symbolic factors such as ordination. Because it confers sacramental authority, interpretive authority, and, in some bodies, decision-making authority, ministerial certification is one significant aspect of pastoral power. Since one aspect of the *contradictory class location* of clergy consists in having an authority or credential that is scarce, religious ordination can be this kind of valued skill. This is the *symbolic* side of pastoral power. It is Foucault's primary emphasis. One way to see pastoral power at work is to imagine how a person who is a minister in a community is immediately accorded respect. The minister is seen as an authority by virtue of calling and not because of how they do their work.

Third, the final aspect of pastoral power has to do with the extent of shared experience and knowledge that a pastoral leader has with a community. As Emmanuel Lartey has argued, every form of pastoral care is intercultural care, since each pastoral care action involves interactions between persons from various cultural groups.[26] The more points of connection the minister has to members of the community, the more likely the minister will have pastoral power in a given scenario. In terms of shared experience, social class can also provide a background from which ministers can understand people in their communities and thus provide more effective care.

Pastoral power *refers to the capacity to lead people and help them interpret their lives. It is a power that comes from the interlocking sources of established trust, symbolic authority, and shared heritage.* Such power can be deployed to address the core conditions of capitalism in which people are being oppressed. Clergy should use their *contradictory class location,* being a professional responsible for valued skills but also close to the working class, to foster solidarity with congregants that can lead to their liberation.

Persons of faith frequently ask about the significance of their lives, their purpose, dignity, and the meaning of their lives with their minister. When they do so ministers have the power to help them interpret their lives. One congregant who could not get a job reached out to a long-time minister and asked "Is there something wrong with me?" Ministers in this position have the privilege of helping people interpret their economic suffering in ways that do not blame the individual. In pastoral power, as opposed to pastoral counseling, the emphasis is on how the community and the individual's story are connected. When congregants reach out to a minister for help, it is often because they are exercising some combination of pastoral power (time travelled with people that lead to earned trust, symbolic authority, and shared cultural location) that helps a minister be seen as a trustworthy arbiter of the faith and an interpreter of people's lives.

At the same time, it is essentially a theological view of the person that undergirds the ways that ministers will interpret the lives of those who seek their help. Ministers believe that there is more to a person's identity than their wealth. As we saw in the previous chapter, pastors typically see people who come to them for care as being created in the Image of God and with a sense of purpose in their lives.

In chapter 3 I told the story of Jim and described how one minister had offered him the keys to the church and a job of sexton for $15 a week. Jim experienced this as a tremendous gift and a statement of inclusion and trust in his journey. Not only had the church given him a job, but also they had trusted him with their sacred space. Yet Jim was already a member of the body of Christ, and he was, in a sense, being hospitable to the church by sharing his gifts and ministry with them. This lead to Jim becoming affiliated with not only that minister's church, but also with a variety of churches and synagogues in the community, giving back his time through assisting the community and caring for them. Pastoral power includes the ability to confer dignity and respect, to thank persons and bless them; it also includes the ability to receive a blessing, to be offered hospitality, and to be transformed.

Given the title of this book and the juxtaposition of pastoral power to psychiatric power as described in chapter 2, ministers are fortunate not to be responsible for the medical diagnosis of emotional suffering, and instead be able to offer a distinctive emerging perspective. Their distance from biological psychiatry gives them a critical distance through which to evaluate the current economic times and the psychological impact of these times.

Resisting the limits of the psy-complex, such as methodological individualism, ministers can engage in a psychology of everyday experience that links the micro-world to the macro-social context. The demands of this work mean that clergy are always holding the one and the many together, as Foucault noted, and this gives the clergy interpretive possibilities. They can see what the individuals in their community are going through in the context of the broader society.

Pastoral power can be used to help foster c/s/x voices in a religious community rather than professional mental health voices alone. In this book we emphasize the socially caused nature of emotional suffering, highlighting c/s/x activist's own testimonies rather than exclusively a biomedical model, and offer advocacy approaches that address some important and neglected causes of psychic suffering. By making this interpretation, ministers can experience a new form of solidarity with persons who come to them seeking emotional help, and this solidarity will help the minister use their pastoral power more effectively with the person in their care. Take for example the phenomenon of mental distress, since many persons with mental suffering come to talk to their clergy. Some people focus on how they have caused their own mental suffering and this self-blame includes religious components, such as the fear of having committed the "unpardonable sin" (Mk. 3:29).[27] In this situation a minister can respond with compassion, indicating both solidarity and an understanding of the factors that contribute to mental distress. Pastoral power is indeed real, and it is a power that is constituted by a combined temporal element—the duration of one's journey with another, the symbolic authority that comes from being a religious leader, and the extent of cultural similarity and difference.

Counter-Conducts of Pastoral Power

Foucault noted the problems that occur when the state takes over the realm of pastoral power and intervenes in the lives of individuals. Fundamentally, he was concerned that pastoral power could be an unfortunate sort of clericalism. He proposed in its place certain "counter-conducts" of pastoral power that would help give people authority through a direct relationship with God and community. Returning people to discover their own authority in the religious realm, these counter-conducts—*mysticism, community, asceticism, Scripture,* and *eschatology*—did not discredit religious power but distributed it differently. Most importantly, the power of religious faith belonged to the community rather than to its ordained leaders.

Religious authority has always been a contested form of authority. He notes that these struggles took place on a variety of fronts that included economic and gender elements. Such deeply impacted a society in which civil and religious order was so closely bound together, in the case of infant baptism, citizenship, and military service. We could say that the counter-conducts relativize pastoral power. By extension, they show that it is necessary to put religious power in the hands of our communities in order to allow transformation to occur.

Foucault was fundamentally suspicious of pastoral power, and with good reason. The potential for abuse of ministerial authority is widespread and becoming increasingly known.[28] Foucault argued that pastoral power was best expressed by the laity themselves through a series of counter-conducts that challenged the limits of clericalism. These counter-conducts were meant for the people, an expression of their faith in God and the extent of their social power. At the heart of the counter-conducts of pastoral power is a shift toward how each person is in a unique relationship with God as an individual and through community. In his historical retrieval of counter-conducts as Christian practices,

Foucault anticipated that utilizing these religious powers could challenge interconnected oppressions of sexism and militarism.[29]

Although Foucault listed the counter-conducts in the following order—asceticism, community, mysticism, Scripture, and eschatology, I shift them into my own order that indicates a priority on my part. In what follows, I briefly illustrate Foucault's concept of each counter-conduct and bring it into conversation with the analysis of social class in an era of neoliberalism. Focusing on the distinctive relationship between God and individuals in community, the counter-conducts have the power to radically relativize our given notions of authority.

Mysticism

Mysticism is the practices of contemplation in which the soul deepens in its relationship with God. As such, mysticism is always in a dialectic with language, meaning that the mystic always deals with the reduction of her experiences with God as she tries to express them in discourse. Likewise, mysticism is always in conversation with the communal and social world, so that the private retreat in which one has spiritual experiences is often the moment when the outside world begins to crowd into one's thoughts. This personal element to religion can be practiced as the presence of God, the assurance of one's faith, prayers of examen, or other forms of spiritual awareness.

In my definition, mysticism has to do with the subjective element of relationship with God in which the soul is confirmed in God's presence. Mysticism should be seen as on a continuum with more traditional and public religious life. Mysticism is not true while organized public religion is false. Rather, mysticism has to do with the direct confirmation of the worth of even the most marginalized.

Foucault argued that mysticism was a direct vulnerability that implied knowledge of God and awareness of God's personal relationship with the soul. "In mysticism the soul sees itself. It sees itself in God and sees God in itself."[30] By definition, mysticism cannot be taught. "In mysticism there is an immediate communication that may take the form of a dialogue between God and the soul, of appeal and response, of the declaration of God's love of the soul, and the soul's love of God."[31] There is no greater knowledge that one can have about the soul than the notion that the soul is known by God, in communication with God, and loved by God.

Jim, whose story I referred to earlier in the chapter, is a c/s/x survivor who redefined his experience of mental distress as inverse paranoia, the conviction that people wanted to do him good. The beginning of Jim's faith was, quite dramatically, when he was sedated for his first of 160 shock treatments. He described crying out to God before his first shock treatment and experiencing God's presence with him for the first time in his life. Since then, he has become a person of profound faith who believes that his journey of emotional suffering has actually been for his own good, a belief that he says he developed through years of relationship with persons in the church.

He noted that when he quieted his soul, he could settle down and experience God's presence. Shaped by his time travelling with the Quakers, he believed in God's unconditional love that met people where they are, regardless of their capacities. Nowadays when he experienced God's presence, it is as a "warm sensation" that tells him everything is going to be fine. Invited up to share his story with the congregation, the minister allowed this counter-conduct of pastoral power to show forth into his community.

In a neoliberal era persons are judged to have worth based on what they can achieve on an individual basis. Those struggling with emotional difficulties are expected to become invisible. Mysticism cuts short this marginalization and reinstates each person as deserving of worth, by confirming before God and others the worthiness of the self regardless of the self's capacities. Jim's story contradicts many themes of a neoliberal economy. He critiques his own job as a dishwasher, stating, "Here's the American dream for you." People who have suffered from emotional distress often feel as if they have worth only if they behave or take medications and are silent. By contrast, mysticism offers a non-capacity oriented picture of the person that sees how each individual is the recipient of a unique truth and a source of Divine knowledge. An individual person is deserving of dignity and respect, not because of what they can earn but because of who they are. God has been present to them, communicating directly to them even if God's communications have been discredited by the wider society. As the c/s/x survivor I quoted in chapter 3 stated, "It was a bit of cheek to arrest me for talking about God."[32]

Mysticism consists in the direct experience of being known and seen by God, and it is completely separate from forms of social control, in which the knowledge of God must be fitted into systems of legitimation. As we can see, language is a difficulty here since it is essentially impossible to put mysticism into language without some loss, transposition, or even violence done to the experience in the process of putting it into words.

As we have seen, the counter-conduct of pastoral power described as *mysticism* is different from a rational proposition: it is more like an affective experience. It is the kind of experience that can heal shame, including social-class shame, but it can be difficult to instantiate for others if one has not experienced it for oneself. Lived mysticism radically unbinds fear and the new reality experienced through it has the potential to become more important than any other mental illness identity. Disability theologian John Swinton tells a story about being approached after a speech at a conference by someone who told him, "I learned from you today that my identity as a Christian is more important than my identity as [someone who has] bipolar."[33] Being seen and known by God became more important than how his psychiatrist saw him.

Even though mysticism is by definition beyond human control, there are also ways that people can bring mysticism into their lives. A small group meeting at a church to talk about their own experiences of emotional suffering in the new economy began with this question, inspired by the counter-conduct of mysticism.

"Imagine that you see yourself in God. What is it like? What do you notice there? How does it feel to you?"

The questions continue, "Imagine that you see God in yourself. What happens in your body? How do you sense this presence?"

Alternatively, in counseling one minister began by asking the parishioner to write briefly on this question: "What would God say to declare God's love to you? How would you declare your love back to God?" For people who have been marginalized, diagnosed, and controlled, these questions can serve to reorient the spirit. Reflecting on them for some time leads to increasing self-gentleness, a rise in respect in one's own eyes, and a perceptible reduction in shame. This indirect healing for a neoliberal era allows the channels of the Spirit to remain open so that persons sees themselves as a center of authority rather than deferring religious authority to another. In this way, people learn of their own significance before God.

The logic of mysticism presumes that God has already been at work in the life of another and seeks to confirm that witness and that presence, noting the worth of the other and also how the other is a central site of authority. Hearing the voice of God in the community of faith requires hearing each other's voices.

Community

Community is a name for that reality through which people in religious life begin to have authority and importance in our own lives. It refers to how we experience our stories as linked to the stories of others, and how we come to be seen and known by them. Community is not the opposite of mysticism in that one would stress sociality while the other would stress individuality. It refers to that reality that the body of believers is always more stable, enduring, and more significant than any given leader. Community is put into place when people begin to pray for one another, when they hear each other's stories and take them to heart, and when they sacrifice for each other, learning from each other's narratives. Community is the name for the linked faith and trust that come from shared experience in which the story of another is no longer seen as belonging only to that person, but also impacts the self. Community has a topsy-turvy element, in that it is often the most vulnerable and marginalized members of a community that offer hospitality to the others. Community is different than a mirror that simply confirms the self, but it is rather a relationship of shared responsibility and mutuality that exists across difference.

In his book *Resurrecting the Person: Friendship with Persons with Mental Illness,* John Swinton tells the story of David, who attends a religious community's small group study after being released from the psychiatric hospital, and he describes the community's reaction:

> They came to understand him as a person who, while at times almost completely obscured by a particularly unpleasant mental health problem, was at other times a person who not only needed to be cared for, *but also cared for them* and enjoyed their company.[34]

The emphasis here is on how people who have suffered from emotional stress, people in working-class positions who face the trials of living in the new economy, care for the church. This means that we move beyond the idea that the community welcomed David, and explore how he welcomed them.

As a member of the body of Christ, David was a central person in the rites and communion of his religious group, a place where he offered radical hospitality to those around him. Thankfully this group responded to his call for community. When he stood up and spoke, interrupting a religious service a few weeks later, this small group was able to advocate for him and help interpret his actions to the entire community.

In order to make community a reality across difference, it is important for people to be educated about the realities of emotional suffering in our neoliberal times. This is important so that people do not misunderstand each other's suffering. What if this small group had been educated in the significant economic factors that play into the inception and course of mental illness, so that they began to understand how the most unequal societies have the highest prevalence of mental illness and the lowest rates of recovery? If this community began to see how social class was related to mental illness, they could begin to advocate, not doing simply "charity" work that provided a one-time uplift, but advocate to shift the conditions that contribute to David's suffering and the whole community's suffering. Community moves from otherness to solidarity.

Foucault gives several examples of communities that have become more interdependent. In these communities, persons often form relationships of mutual responsibility that become more important than official religious authority. In the Taborites, for example, a minister does not have any defining characteristic, but only some responsibilities for a time, with no sacramental role.[35] Other communities continue the sacramental tradition, but decouple this institution from civil and legal roles, as in the Anabaptist's rejection of infant baptism and thus citizenship and military conscription.[36] Even communities who do not have clergy instill a sense of shared responsibility among themselves. In one community, two friends made a covenant of obedience to one another, offering to honor one another's commandment as if they were the commandments of God—they kept this covenant for 28 years.[37] While vows of religious obedience often instill this kind of serious commitment, it is unusual to find it among friends.

Community has to do with shared relationship and shared responsibility for one another rather than depending on pastoral leadership alone. The significance of obedience to one minister is subsumed into the new relationships of shared obedience in community.

What is at stake here is a theological claim. Christian community involves empathic identification and also something more. Christian community is one in which the needs of another do not simply put a demand on a person. Neither does the presence of another simply add something beneficial. Rather, by being in community with one another, people become substantially new selves as they hear one another's stories in the religious sphere, both sharing one another's burdens but also being constituted intersubjectively by practices of relating to one another.

The community that forms around one another's stories also has a class location. It is processing the avoidable suffering that comes from times of vast economic inequality and inhuman working conditions. Thus the stories that are shared also have to do with one's labor, how it is procured from one, and also what it takes to be in a relationship with other laborers. In one community a congregation put together a community-based organizing group who responded when neighbors were at risk for foreclosure. In one case, 20 congregants drawn from multiple parishes and faith communities, gathered to pray for Juan, a man facing foreclosure. This man was finally able to get a loan modification and refinance his home so he could stay in it. The advocacy of his religious community prevented untold emotional suffering in his life. Given what we learned about the contribution of home foreclosure to mental illness in entire communities, this is a way of addressing mental health concerns in communities preemptively.

As Jonathan Tran argued in his book on *Foucault and Theology*, it is "God's giving of his own body that makes capitalistic notions of property, scarcity and competition, literal privations of the good."[38] Since community means participating in God's body, even worship becomes a site of resistance against the dominance of a capital-based vision of the human person.[39]

Asceticism

The extent to which we are shaped by the market and the incitement to wealth and advantage means that there is little room at times for the kinds of solidarity in which one could identify with the suffering of others. Foucault indicates that asceticism as a sort of self-chosen suffering cuts across the limits of pastoral power by not being afraid of suffering and, indeed, seeing suffering as part of Christ's suffering.

In this section I take a different approach from Foucault, whose discussion of asceticism previews some of his later discussion of sexuality in the Greco-Roman period. Foucault is interested in asceticism for its own sake. As such, while obedience seeks to manage and control the suffering, Foucault considered asceticism as a sort of experiment that fell outside the control of obedience. He highlights how ascetics often link their suffering with the suffering of Christ.

What I am most interested in is how asceticism can be used in *contradictory class locations* to help persons foster solidarity with those in the working class. In chapter 1, I showed how ministers are compensated for their skills and credentials but how they often hold a financial position closer to those whom they serve. This is because they are in the "comfort" class, essentially working class because they are not able to save or invest. The kind of asceticism we are discussing here is the use of one's own class and social power to alleviate another's needless suffering, all the while refusing to see that other as deserving of pity or charity. Granting that we all have "the market" inside us to some extent, we are tempted to glorify and implicitly identify with the rich, seeing money as an end itself.[40] Grappling with asceticism could be similar to what Rieger describes as transforming our desire, a lengthy process.[41]

Thus, I do not see the kind of avoidable suffering we have been discussing in chapter 1 as an end in itself but as a reality on the way to transformation. Such suffering should build awareness of another's experience and allegiances with that other in order to transform that unnecessary suffering. Joerg Rieger has argued that this transformation means deconstructing how one's images of God have become unconsciously connected to theological power and wealth and instead identifying with Jesus the Christ who was incarnated as a day laborer.

Because financial suffering impacts so much of a person's psychic and emotional life, asceticism also involves crucial forms of interpretation to help persons become liberated: namely, resisting the internal attribution of suffering for factors that are inherently socially caused and mediated. Resisting the stigma of being in a working-class position is also connected to addressing the stigma of mental illness. Interpreting suffering rightly means shifting the focus to those things that continue to cause suffering and being *ascetic* about our own identity labels. This means resisting the terms that obscure people's suffering.

Communities may already be facing so many struggles that it can be difficult to expect them to be ascetic. Nevertheless, the greater the financial resources, the greater necessity there is for communities to engage in asceticism for others in their vicinity. For example, a wealthy suburban congregation decided to postpone a building project on a Christian Education wing for their church and instead began a day program that helped laborers in a nearby inner-city community to find work. This partnership became a way that this congregation could become ascetic.

Scripture

The minister who gathers a group for Scripture study suddenly realizes that three of its members are unemployed and a fourth has been fired recently, and she turns the group to a discussion of the Gospels where Jesus takes compassion on the crowd because they are "harassed" like sheep without a shepherd (Mt. 9:36). Opening the question of what this means, she sets the frame for the conversation but lets the group share their thoughts.

Foucault notes that Scripture is at the heart of the counter-conducts of pastoral power. The ability of believers to interpret Scripture for themselves, and the confirmation of authority through this interpretation, is one of the primary ways that believers had of accessing an awareness of God's presence—the kind described in mysticism.

Both Protestants and Catholics confirm the importance of Scriptures as God's authoritative revelation, and that it is also a narrative of God's presence with a particular people. Here we offer this interpretive principle to best allow the counter-conduct of Scripture to be useful in community.

The texts of Scripture proclaim God's blessing on those who actively work to alleviate the suffering of the poor, and so our own interpretations of Scripture should be geared toward this same end. The frame in which the story of the church has unfolded is one in which God's radical mercy crossed-class relationships, establishing new forms of solidarity in communities in which persons were seen as unworthy, as invisible, and even as shameful.

Indeed, we could say that Scripture provides such communities a sense of themselves, so that interpreting Scripture in communities such as these becomes a faithful way of attending to God's own presence. This interpretive community for Scripture reveals working-class concerns, namely the primacy of God's liberation of oppressed people, and also refocuses them on tasks of interpretation. For example, redaction criticism and other technical matters can be subsumed to the fundamental goal of liberation.

Feminist scholars have been exploring ways of expanding the interpretive framework—Letty Russell and Lucy Rose have each proposed models of shared interpretation that open up the task of understanding the Scriptures to the whole community.[42] When this happens, working-class concerns enter the framework. The goal of communal understanding of economic suffering becomes crucial to the interpretation of Scripture in our era in order for working-class persons to feel as if God cares about them. Scripture can be used to orient one's imagination to the plight of the excluded classes, as well as challenges to the work of liberation.

There are interpretive mistakes that communities can make in their understanding of Scripture, one of the worst of which has to do with the financialization of God's promises, the excesses of a popular text such as the "Prayer of Jabez," a book based upon a Biblical allusion that promised increased wealth.[43] These excesses involve a fundamental misunderstanding of the intended aim and audience of Scripture.

A way that communities can shape their engagement with Scripture is by asking "How would working class persons experience God's presence with them and advocacy for them through these texts?" Further, "How would such a text lead to the transformation of conditions that lead to suffering, wage theft, and other concerns?" A further step involves actually including the voices of the dispossessed in this process. Avaren Ipsen's insightful book of Scripture interpretation with sex workers is one helpful example.[44]

The interpretation of Scripture is conflicted and always grounded in a particular group's interest. In this case I am arguing that the primacy of c/s/x activists concerns and worker's rights movements coalesce around a liberating interpretation of the Bible. The study of the Bible, when it is extended beyond its typical hermeneutics of privilege, becomes a part of the struggle of people for just living conditions and rights. These questions also provide a framework within which to struggle with some of the disturbing aspects of Scripture, for example how it contributes to the oppression of women and seems to countenance slavery in some of its pages.[45] When Scripture is oriented toward liberation, seeing the subject of Scripture as those who have been oppressed, then it becomes clearer how Scripture can be used in community to foster cross-class solidarity.

Eschatology

Persons from working-class positions tend to believe more strongly in eschatological themes such as heaven or hell, a personal God or devil. These very elements are often deconstructed through theological education.[46] Yet, the promise of Christian theology's eschatology is that it indicates a final horizon of human meaning—people do not simply make choices based on their financial interests or what benefits them, but there is a broader horizon of God's justice against which human decisions will be placed.

Of course, Christian eschatology must also avoid an exclusive otherworldliness. Recent works in eschatology have emphasized a *realized eschatology* and not the impact that our thinking about "last things" has on our present. The primary means of eschatology is the hope that God's justice will be revealed in ways that restore right relationships, and it is this hope that provides energy for the continued efforts of justice. Note that the counter-conduct of eschatology is more than a Marxist historical materialism in which a new classless society provides the end toward which all our efforts are directed. Lest it risk naïve otherworldliness, even Christian eschatology must grapple with the conditions of neoliberal capitalism.

Foucault describes how eschatology revises all pastoral power, and his description underlines the limited and fallible nature of all ministries. "The times are being fulfilled or in the process of being fulfilled, and that God will return or is returning to gather his flock. He will be the true shepherd."[47] Note the importance of the language of nourishment. Dreaming of justice and longing for God's reign, so that spiritual and material realities are overlapping and connected.

People live under tremendous pressure, and praying "Come, Lord Jesus" along with the first Christian communities are proclaiming something more than a panacea that covers over social injustice. It is a way of being faithful to God that does not erase the conditions of everyday suffering in which people so often feel trapped, but it still makes a difference. Indeed, eschatology can be a profound source of energy, a true counter-conduct, redirecting pastoral power as it releases the notion of the status quo and energizes people with a vision that the present is not all that there is.

On the other hand, the faith of otherworldly revivalism, if it does not have an element of critique of the existing social order, serves to strengthen the bonds of injustice. In her book *Nickel and Dimed*, Barbara Ehrenreich discusses how she attended a tent revival meeting when she was working a series of low-wage jobs in South Florida. The revival preachers all emphasized how people were indebted to Jesus for his death for them.[48] There was no mention of the life of Jesus and his works of healing and ministry. She urged the Christian community to retrieve themes from Jesus Christ's earthly ministry, not simply his death, so that working-class people could experience liberation.

The themes of liberation can be seen if eschatology becomes effective in communities. Such projects for practical eschatology include the reclamation of the notion of a Jubilee year in which the land is allowed to rest. Modern Christian churches have argued that wealthy nations use this principle to relieve the debt burden of poorer nations. Indeed, in his sermon in Galilee where he teaches in the synagogue, Jesus states that he has come to instantiate the year of Jubilee, the relationship of indebtedness being transformed (Deut. 15:12).

What is crucial is that eschatology be seen not as providing an erasure of the violence of human history, but rather as fulfilling the claims of the oppressed on their oppressors. Directly addressing these economic conditions is one way that the principle of eschatology can be made real.

In this counter-conduct, people inspired by eschatology do not invalidate the importance of the environment or the actual world in which we live. Rather, they are inspired by the conditions of justice to change the circumstances of the environment, fostering a more sustainable future. In what follows I explore in a more poetic fashion what the counter-conducts of pastoral power mean in community, by crafting some concluding remarks on the complex and contradictory nature of pastoral power.

Ministry—a Complex Justice

Ministers are almost the last people you would expect to feel powerful. Living in homes owned by others on the outskirts of society, destined to drive cheap cars with a better world ahead, ready with a word and a smile, an offer of help, a box of nails, a prayer.

Ministers are almost the last people you would expect to have power. Called up at the last minute to cut a ribbon, bless a baby, a marriage, called in the middle of the night to hospital to witness the dissolution of a dream, ministers are nearly powerless.

The daily life of ministry is pockmarked with mediocrity, cross-hatched with the care of committees and renovations, keeping the doors open or trying to get there on time, caring with all your soul and grief and yet wondering if you care too much. It means caring about all the small-time cares.

A seminary graduate works at a downtown homeless shelter and opens the church as a sanctuary for the poor. They shuffle in, mumbling to themselves at times. She knows one man who is trying to get workman's compensation because his legs were shattered from a fall at work. He's been increasingly sad. He used to have a lot of theories about what went wrong in his life. Now he's mostly silent except in prayer, "I shall not want," and then again, "give us this day our daily bread."

Profound conditions of helplessness, speechless terror, longing for justice, singing Psalms of lament and comfort, ministers live in the daily rhythm of work and rest with people, knitting their lives together with communion and care.

There is no ministry apart from life. Pull at the strands—friendship, food, family—and out come all the other complexities, despair, compulsion, regret, fear. Justice does not breathe the reified air of the best of all possible worlds. It travels here below, through transportation struggles, in and out of disability, via nights and days of unimaginable pain, along with strikes and protests, through opaque nights of the soul. All this happens in the middle of the liturgical year, in ordinary time.

Ministers are among the least powerful people. The pastorate takes place in the midst of life, not in a privileged time warp. A minister leans in to listen because she believes Another is listening. She cares and counsels with a *"Third presence"* in the room. She leads liturgies in street protests with the working class because she believes in God's final justice. She celebrates and officiates and preaches from the prophets, hoping for a world to live up to, to believe with again. She prays *"Come, Lord Jesus"* like the heroes of the faith that have inspired her.

The Invitation to Ministry

In the earlier discussion, I indicated the narrow scope of power ministers have, yet my writing indicated that there still *was* a form of pastoral power, veiled as it seemed under the cloak of the common and in the dress of the everyday. On the one hand, pastoral power frequently begins with an invitation, such as Jesus Christ's invitation to "Come and see" (Jn. 1:39). People often invite us to come and see the conditions and circumstances of their lives. At times, this invitation is explicit, and at other times it is circumstantial, and even in this invitation to witness, ministers may not completely understand what they are invited to see. When a hospice chaplain enters a home to find the house strewn with bottles, he knows he is a stranger to a certain pain. When a minister is shooed away from the door of a man who has been experiencing discouragement for several weeks, she knows the ambiguity of this role.

Yet sometimes the invitation to ministry appears more like a demand: a woman is seeking shelter from an abusive husband, the state calls to see if the church would host children from Honduras who need a place to stay while the state seeks services. The world is at one's doorstep in a way that seems to prevent the luxury of reflection.

An invitation, a demand, a call to witness: an immediate call for response to an action that will have ethical consequences and be interpreted by an entire community or world. Pastoral figures bear witness in ordinary time through care for imperfect institutions that they hope can do the most good. They care through the complexities of life in concrete actions and in language that they borrow for liturgy, Scripture, and proclamation. They care through executive summaries and reports that break down the experience of intense social suffering into a form that can be more readily understood so that the good work can go on. At times they break. At other times they break the rules—helping out the contingent class for the greater good.

Action and language belong together in ministry. At times simply showing up is a profound testimony. In other circumstances a word is called for, a word that approaches the prophetic, so that justice can be done, victims will not be blamed but believed, and God will be worshipped more faithfully. Action is a form of language—hands held and prayer sung at the courthouse go on the nightly news and now everyone knows "where the minister stands." Language is a form of action—"God bless you." "Hear the Good news." It is not simply that actions speak louder than words but that word and action speak together in the context of a world that is suffering tremendously.

The primary context of ministry is a world where people cannot make ends meet and where the working class are stigmatized for their difficulties. Ministry gains its perspective from listening to this suffering and seeing it, not turning away and looking the other direction. The concerns of the working-class persons laboring outside the church need to be in the foreground of our pastoral imagination. All too often the everyday concerns of middle or upper class professional life grab the attention of the church. This is frequently a church that has left the city for the suburbs. Yet there is a widespread fear that must be attended to in these times, a fear that ends may not meet, and that, if money is all we are, we might just add up to nothing in the end.

Listening as Prayer: Prayer as Listening

When I visited the hospital room of a psychiatric patient who believed in Urantia, a new US religious group with a belief in personal divinity and a developed cosmology, I listened to his whole story. At the end, the patient said, "Thank you for listening," and there was a long pause where we locked eyes. He was a spark of the Divine.

I turned to the patient's psychiatric file and found a complex history, but the words failed to capture the person I had just heard. When the patient threw a table and broke its legs later that week, I could intervene so that he was not placed in restraints. As I talked in the hallway I was listening to him and believing him.

As Bonhoeffer says "the first service believers owe to one another is listening to them."[49] In his book *The Presence of God in Pastoral Counseling* Wayne Oates suggests that Christ is the "Third Presence" in pastoral care and counseling, which means that attentive listening is an act of prayer.[50] I submit that prayer is the noninstrumental vehicle through which the counter-conducts become an effective exercise of pastoral power. Prayer and listening belong together in pastoral care and counseling.

Through attentive listening one attends to Christ, which is a political act. Yet Christ is hidden in our midst, as transformed as in the sacrament. Listening with attention to the presence of Christ is not an add-on to the practice of listening. Through the eyes of faith it becomes the conceptual core of listening and prayer, since Christ takes on the strangest of forms.

In this book I argue that emotional distress and working-class concerns should be high on the agenda of pastoral ministers and I imply that ministers have something distinctive to give that is not encapsulated by biomedical psychiatry. In chapter 3 we saw how one of the chief desires of persons with emotional distress was simply someone to reach out to when they felt troubled. Ministers play this role when they listen to and pray with persons in their midst who are struggling with emotional distress.

Yet ministers also need to see the distressed in their midst who may never attend their worship. Union activists in the Dallas area struggled to get clergy to hear their concerns.[51] In this book I maintain that in listening to the testimony of those suffering we become, in Cresswell's terms drawn from chapter 3, a *partner* to it. Ministers also pray when they hear someone's story, turning everyday acts of care into political tasks for justice and faith and praying for God's ultimate justice in the face of unbelievable pain.

What does it mean, then, to pray, an act that is often conceived as the heart of pastoral work? Prayer cannot be understood as an episodic event. It is not a means toward the end of well-being. It does not occur exclusively in private or in public. Prayer is not set apart from power in the realm of the spiritual. It *is* an act of power, done by one who makes promises to One whose promises are trustworthy.[52] It is not an achievement or a duty, a formal trick to end pastoral conversations. It is instead the only hope of the soul struggling for hope against hope. Prayer with those who are suffering from emotional distress, prayer with the working class, are each struggles for justice with God.

Prayer is an act of listening that begins and ends often after formal prayer. It occurs in the depths and the heights and echoes of the voices of the deceased. Through prayer we gain solidarity with those who can no longer speak, whose voices are silenced by suffering and injustice, by psychic pain and different forms of ability.[53] Prayer is primarily an act of listening taken on in the body that connects us across time and speechlessness.

Prayer occurs in relationship with God and is the fulfillment of human speech, as well as all of our speechless cries. It is in prayer within our traditions that we curse our enemies, that we pray for deliverance, and that we long for a sustainable future. Prayer is an act of listening to a centuries-old past, a past in which God has chosen a ravaged people and set up a home among them, a temporary dwelling place that can be moved, so that God acknowledges all their specificity, their blessedness, their petty hatreds, their mundane cares.

It is indeed only prayer that enables us to keep faith with God in the presence of tremendous suffering and injustice. The capacity of prayer to hold us together allows a double focus to emerge—a focus on systemic injustice and a focus on personal meaning. Greed from corporate capitalism and the suffering that comes from depression. Gentrification in the inner city and the particular man who began shouting in the street in the middle of the night because he was displaced.

Prayer keeps us awake to suffering and enables us to see the context of a person. No longer must we numb out to avoid the feelings of hopelessness. Indeed, we have companions for ourselves on this journey. *The church is the sum of all stories of suffering, told and untold, under the sign of the cross, and its ecclesial shape is prayer.* As we can see, distinction between private prayer and public worship destabilize as we link practice and speech.

Conclusion

In this chapter I explore the distinctive impact of pastoral power in the condition of neoliberalism, tracing the significant symbolic authority of ministry but also offering the counter-conducts as the fulfillment of pastoral power. A central theme of this chapter is how the entire ministry can be shaped around people's own experience of God's presence with them and the importance of community in that presence.

When ministers operate in close connection with psy-complex, they gain expertise in psychological interventions. But they also gain a certain view of the world, one in which the illness model comes to the fore. As we note in chapter 2, the medicalization of our feelings continue apace in a neoliberal era and ministers sometimes represent these ways of thinking uncritically. This can lead to a diminishment of their own theological perspectives, even as they may gain legitimacy in the psychological counseling sphere.

Other clergy feel that they lack the distinctive tools to help their communities struggling through the economic downturn, and they turn to psychologists, social workers, and psychiatrists to help. These can be significant sources of support.

In this chapter I explore the significance of the counter-conducts as the gift of the people for revitalizing faith and challenging injustice. Seen in a variety of forms, it is that essential character of communion in which the vulnerable create relationships of care with another. Yet is also the hope of liberation from injustice, so that people can fully bring their faith to bear on the circumstances of their suffering. Of course, this takes a great deal of cross-class solidarity, people articulating in their own voices their vision for what matters to them.

In this chapter I also offer in a more poetic style the interconnected complexity of ministry in the face of injustice, emphasizing prayer. I note how the everyday rituals of ministry link up with experiences of class oppression and mental suffering. In this chapter I indicate how the complex acts of ministry are responses to the demands of justice and invitations to become a partner to person's stories. From this vantage point, the personal and the structural are linked in the form of language-acts that occurs in pastoral ministry, and the church is seen as the living form of all these connected acts, culminating in the people's gracious vision of God.

In chapter 6 we explore how the church can more completely instantiate its reality as a cross-class society that attends to the injustice caused by the new economy and the mental suffering that has resulted. Summing up the themes of the book, chapter 6 clearly describes what is at stake in turning the working class into psychiatric patients. I interpret the struggles of the Corinthian community as revolving around cross-class dynamics in their community, and I suggest how the counter-conducts of pastoral power can be used to more consciously foster solidarity across class lines, with the goal of addressing the avoidable suffering of living within a highly classed society. If we have seen how we must attend to the most silenced stories, having a preferential option for these, we then see how to foster church life so that silenced stories are not forgotten.

CHAPTER 6

An Integrative Vision for Pastoral Power

At a small church in an inner-city storefront in a community that has undergone massive factory closures, a pastor preaches about unemployment. Afterward, she gathers in a circle with parishioners for prayer, lifting their concerns up for the church to hear and praying together to God. Here is something more than a panacea or the opiate of the people. The minister does not simply sanctify the situation as it is, but focuses on how the community can continue on in the face of adversity. The minister in prayer brings together the chief concerns of the whole person, its soul and its survival, and removes any doubt that this suffering is in any way the fault of these individuals.

In my argument I maintain that pastoral care and counseling must take into account the economic factors that shape people's identities and experiences, rather than simply the interpersonal themes relating to family life that have been the traditional focus of pastoral care. Most forms of oppression are two-dimensional in that they involve both recognition—for example struggles around racial or gender equality—*and* redistribution.[1] As we have seen in this text, economic oppression itself is frequently multidimensional, in that it involves both the recognition of marginalized identities and the widespread need for redistribution.

Neoliberalism has been explored as a central cultural frame in this book, namely the discourse of private rights and market dominance that has occurred in the last 40 years. It was based in a philosophy of trickle-down economics, the notion that a few wealthy persons could spread universal good to all. This form of implicit faith has been one of the driving ideologies of our time. As we have seen, the good given to a few has not led to benefits for all, and this philosophy has even clouded our thinking—it has spawned a glorification of the owning class and a denigration of the working class. At times this divide has received theological legitimacy, as persons have tended to identify God with the attributes of power that come from money.[2] At other times the theological legitimation has been subtler, as in avoiding the topic of economics altogether in religious space.

In this very season in which so much emphasis has been placed on wealth, with so little to go around, people are vulnerable to stigmatizing language that puts the blame on them for factors that are cultural in nature. A central issue in the book has been the productive notion of discourse drawn from Michel Foucault: the combination of both the rules and regulations and the institutions that source them. Discourse is more than a prohibition. It is productive speech that covers a person's experience and that shrouds other aspects of their narrative in obscurity.

Exploring the names that have been given to mental distress in our day through biomedical psychiatry, it is clear that the names are inadequate to the forms of suffering under which people labor. Struggling to get enough food to feed their children, much less pay for light and gas, people are wrestling with experiences that are only poorly hinted at through the language of psychopathology. Rather than pointing to disorder, many people suffer from distress, from violated compassion, and the daily degradation of not being seen and heard as a peer in the spaces in which one seeks to be known by others. These kinds of stresses cannot be captured on a list of symptoms from a Diagnostic Manual. They escape from the page into the texture of everyday life. Beyond simply falling short of the complexity of everyday life, psychopharmaceutical logic constructs a person as one who needs to consume to return to the normal level of functioning.

Yet from its inception there have been voices that have challenged both the empirical claims and power practices of psychiatry. They have often done so on an entirely different logical groundwork than the discipline of medicine itself. Instead of replacing the diagnosis with a more accurate one, some have created frameworks that revise existing schema to include richer notions of their experience—their encounters with war, racism, poverty, and God—and positioned their experiences of mental illness as counting as a particular kind of knowledge, a knowledge that cannot be easily dismissed.

This means that along with the constant struggle of poverty, social class also includes the double deprivation of indignity or shame in many instances. Alleviating this shame means directly confronting the neoliberal strategies of shaming—for example, giving degrading names to people who draw from the social safety net that is the common heritage of those who belong to a given society. Resistance in this way also requires alternatives that speak to the release of feeling. Rather than accepting shame, actively resisting social-class shame means telling new stories about the experiences of poverty, sharing these stories openly, and offering a communal revision of the central aspects of our psychology and theology to attend to these forms of distress.

In this book I have argued that in our time it is impossible to address mental illness without also addressing the issue of economic justice, since much of the suffering of our time is avoidable suffering caused by economic factors such as inequity, poor working conditions, and unstable housing or transportation. In that way, addressing the stigma of mental illness is only possible if we focus on another form of stigmatization that also affects many—the stigma of being working class and the cultural perceptions and attributions that are placed on the working- class people. Moving beyond this stigmatizing approach means fostering alliances that craft both self-definition and self-determination within the framework of rights.

Working-Class Suffering in the Church

The disability movement has begun to theorize the importance of access for persons with disabilities as a constituent aspect to the church's identity, arguing that the church cannot be itself unless it is accessible.[3] Persons who suffer from the joint stigma of being in a working-class position and also having emotional distress are frequently denied access from worship as well, and thus not able to engage fully in what it means to be religious persons. Thus, fostering access to worship for the working and contingent class is a central task of accessibility that has to do with church living out its mission.

Stigma-busting approaches to disability often rely on a radical disability model that argues that social disability comes from a lack of access, not from a lack of capacities. When we expand our frameworks to include emotional suffering, we can see that it is not hearing voices that makes one disabled, but rather the lack of access to a normative community that can provide acceptance and resources.

In these times, emotional distress is more widespread than ever before, and much of it is avoidable psychic suffering caused by the economic conditions of our neoliberal era. This means that mental suffering is to some extent socially caused, and that we need to ameliorate that suffering in order to prevent what portion of emotional suffering is related to economic oppression. From this vantage point, it is not merely inclusion of presumed difference (recognition) but also addressing the factors that contribute to suffering (redistribution) that becomes a central part of the pastoral goal.

In order to do this a minister does not have to know what part of mental suffering comes from economic oppression and what is biologically caused, thus dividing the psyche into parts in pastoral counseling. It is enough to know that people suffer unjustly when their work is taken from them, and they are compensated without an adequate means to survive. It also enough to know that much of this suffering shows up as psychic pain that can then lead to disability. If a person becomes disabled due to emotional distress such as severe cases of mental illness, then the radical social model of disability applies—we need to work actively to include them in the body of the faithful so that we can truly be the church God has called us to be. The fact that we are, as a society, responsible for one another's social suffering adds a level of complexity to this task.

As we can see, this is a different aim with different presumptions than one-time charity efforts at the holiday season or soup kitchen work.[4] It means that instead of temporary uplift onto a higher rung on the capitalist order, and instead of glorifying the faith and happiness of the poor—"they have so little, but are so content"—we must risk seeing a different story. We risk seeing how some in society are systematically disadvantaged, and how this is an intentional part of the design of the capitalist system: the disadvantage of one group leads to the profits of another.[5]

Becoming the church in this environment requires challenging deeply held and stereotypical notions about merit that are close to the core of US society, that the poor are somehow different kinds of persons and that the rich somehow deserve their wealth. Facing the facts in churches and counseling spaces shows instead that people are positioned in class arrangements that tend to foster inequity and unjust working conditions. The fact that these class positions remain relatively stable can lead to cynicism, but these conditions can also be shifted through concerted effort, courage, and imagination.

We can see already that this requires something more than simple hospitality or "copious hosting," but it requires a transformation on both sides.[6] Those who have been the beneficiaries of wealth and the power that comes from it need to see such wealth and power not as their right or inheritance. As such, deconstructing the naturalness of wealth means disputing that there are different types of people, the wealthy and the poor. In this way, the working and contingent classes can then be seen as subjects in their own rights, with needs and desires, with names, destinies, and hopes for their future.

Becoming Church in Corinth—the Social Body

A key question that we must face is how can we experience the story of another as implicating us, as calling for a change in our lives, and as directly impacting our own narratives. For persons who are experts and managers, rather than blaming or scapegoating persons in the working class, how is it possible to find that their stories directly impact one's own narratives and are indeed essential to those narratives? In order for this to occur, it is necessary to experience a new understanding of what it means to be linked together in community, a vision that is resourced by the early narratives of the Christian community. All too often, religious institutions seem to legitimate inequality, so that broad-scale studies in Europe and the United States have found that the most unequal societies are also the most religious societies, and that religiosity actually can contribute to inequity.[7] If this is so, then religion may be playing the role of propping up the status quo and may require the refreshment of its emancipatory visions.

In interpreting Scriptures, we should listen for strategies of liberation from ancient texts, and challenge practices within them for how they continue to oppress persons. One set of helpful texts for considering pastoral care in the context of economic oppression is the Corinthian correspondence, which, although it has been oppressive for women since Paul seems to reaffirm gender hierarchy, also challenges the social power of the first century with new models for community.

In this brief discussion of the body metaphor from the Corinthian correspondence, I draw from the socio-scientific study of the New Testament undertaken by scholars Gerd Theissen and Dale Martin, to argue that the Corinthian correspondence's notion of the church as *the body* help us understand something essential about the honor and shame accorded to social class. This new understanding can help us interpret social class today.

Martin maintains that in the Corinthian correspondence Paul is mediating between two factions in the group, the "strong" and the "weak." The strong have, somewhat contradictorily, a philosophy of both Stoic self-restraint and liberality. What seems important is that they are able to exercise their authority over church members who are deemed as "weak" without any perceived consequences.

Martin argues that what we have in the early Corinthian correspondence is a difference between social statuses, not directly corresponding to modern industrial notions of class, but having to do with the social power inherent in relationships. He argues that the strong may have been persons "in the middle area between the true elite and the poor," and the weak were persons whose labor was continuously exploited from them in a fashion that they were seen as *nonpersons* by the surrounding society.[8] Martin summarizes, "What we have in the Corinthian church then, is a division between those who to a great extent controlled their own economic destiny and those who did not."[9] It is within this cross-class context, then, that some of the themes of the Corinthian correspondence come into focus.

Paul famously redefines the Corinthian church as largely coming from the category of *nonpersons,* "Not many of you were wise by human standards, not many were powerful, not many were of noble birth" and he invites the entire church to envision themselves as a body with interdependent parts rather than divided along status lines (1 Cor. 1:26). I envision this metaphor to be a profound and guiding image to bring to life the notion of the community of stories in the previous chapter. Since the church is like a body, interdependent in its various members, it is impossible to break off interest or concern for the working and the excluded classes in the church's midst. It is because of this inherent integrity of the Christian body across social classes that the most silenced stories of suffering in the Christian body must be heard.

> For just as the body is one and has many members, and all the members of the body, though many, are one body, so it is with Christ... The eye cannot say to the hand, "I have no need of you," nor again the head to the feet, "I have no need of you." On the contrary, the members of the body that seem to be weaker are indispensable, and those members of the body that we think less honorable we clothe with greater honor, and our less respectable members are treated with greater respect (1 Cor. 1:12, 21–23).

In this memorable passage Paul evokes the metaphor of the body to call for Christian unity in the Corinthian church. The trope of the body was actually a common theme in ancient literature. Martin notes that this theme was used to reinforce status hierarchies as the head was presumably over the feet as certain social groups were meant to be over others.[10]

Yet, according to Martin, Paul revises the familiar trope of status hierarchies implicit in the body image and reverses them from the inside out. Paul uses the body image to deconstruct given social norms about unity and about appropriate bodies. Through his rhetoric Paul demonstrates that it is actually persons who seemingly have less status that "are actually the most necessary of the body's members."[11] It is not that the church simply reaches out to those of lower social status and thus makes them worthy; rather, it is that the church has fundamentally misunderstood the character and qualities of those who have lower status in their communities and thereby a radical reversal in values takes place. The lower status members in the Corinthian body "have a legitimate claim, therefore, to honor and care from the other body members."[12] Paul deconstructs that status order using a familiar theme from his time that had been used to keep hierarchies in place, for example, just as the head is over the rest of the body you should be in submission to me. In contrast, he argues that our typical notions of status and importance are completely incorrect, thereby dismantling the social status structure upon which the early Christian church was supposedly building its order.

Interpreting the Corinthian metaphors for the body we can see a powerful reversal is taking place that we can use strategically in our own hermeneutics of the church, or what we think of as the human being-in-relationship. We cannot simply draw from Paul a direct blueprint or analogy for our times, but may, through a provocative reading, spin out a set of strategies to help make sense out of our fractured communities. The early Christian church in Corinth seemed to reflect status separations that were seen as a *natural* part of the human order. If we think we know who is more valuable to a given society, Paul confounds this thinking. In the new Christian community he envisions we must temporarily suspend, if not reverse this logic of worth. One of the reasons for this reversal is that in Christ persons of all classes are incorporated into Christ's body. The Corinthian correspondence argues that the given status arrangements are no longer valid in the new society.

In Paul's reading, persons with lower social status were necessary to the church. This means that their distinctive experience of suffering—being seen as having lower social status, being ignored, being discriminated against—were significant and necessary themes to understand the true nature of the church. Rather than being the kinds of experiences that should be shunted to the side and hidden because of some presumed shame, the daily indignities and violations of working-class life, being excluded, of having one's work unfairly extracted, and the mental and emotional suffering that came from the dignity and invisibility of this life, needed to have conceptual and epistemological status at the center of the church's witness.

Our interpretation of the metaphor of the body in the Corinthian correspondence leads us to this conclusion: the church is a collection of stories in which privilege should be given to the most silenced stories. The *nonperson* in the Corinthian community is not meant to be an *object* of the communities care, but that person is also the *subject* within the Corinthian body, of equal worth and integrity in a particular way that may have scandalized members of Paul's readership who were upper class. Fundamental social perceptions prevalent in Paul's time were mistaken because of what it meant to be a body, a new reality that was instantiated through Christ.

Paul insisted that this community already was the body of Christ in the way he described, but we could maintain that it takes real effort to instantiate the community fully in our midst. This means that the stories of working- and excluded-class persons are stories that must impact the self-identity and narratives of the expert- and owning-class persons because these stories implicate who we are in the body of Christ. Reversing social hierarchies in this fashion means placing a priority on the interconnected nature of stories within the Christian community. It is necessary to do works of kindness or charity for persons struggling with poverty and unjust wages in the new economy. A crucial aspect of being an interdependent body as a Christian community in the twenty-first century in the United States is to understand the experiences of people in the working class and excluded class in our midst by giving status and worth to their interpretations and an epistemological privilege—how we know what we claim to know—to their experience.

I submit that the church is a communion of its most silenced stories and that by attending to these narratives we both reflect and instantiate the narrative and sacramental character of the church's life. In the Corinthian correspondence, a reversal of status took place in which Paul deconstructed notions of social worth based on the familiar metaphor of the social body—which in its time had been used to reinforce hierarchies—and argued that the perception of worth and status that were used in his time were limited and must be replaced with new egalitarian notions of honor within the Christian community. I have been applying these categories in order to argue that our narratives are not separated from one another.

As I argued in the previous chapter, *the church is the sum of all stories of suffering, told and untold, and its ecclesial shape is prayer.* Thus church has the potential to give us a different image of the human being, provided it can actualize its countercultural perspective. In order to bring about the reality of such Christian community in the twenty-first century, we must explore our taken-for-granted images of the human being, for example, the image of the successful person or the psychologically healthy individual.

Mental Distress, a Widely Placed Net

Psychopharmaceutical advertising regularly bombards us with images of whether we are mentally healthy enough, combined with class cues that link happiness with middle-class identity.[13] Although this book has argued that there is a kind of suffering that comes from unemployment, problem debt, and foreclosure, it has not, on the other hand, argued that being positioned in the professional or owning class leads to psychic well-being or emotional or spiritual health, for that matter.[14] We are not made healthier by climbing to the top, replacing an economic scale of value with a psychological one.

It is often one's immediate surroundings that mirror back to one the reality of one's social position, confirming or denying one's place in it. That is why in an age of media saturation, when advertising makes us measurably unhappy, there are more people comparing themselves to each other.[15] People at the top such as elite business owner Sean Hanauer have begun to question the super-capitalist system, arguing that redistribution is necessary.[16] Persons such as Hanauer understand that they cannot contribute enough to the social good to compensate for what they are taking from it in income. When they begin to see the suffering caused by massive inequalities and their own role in continuing them, they want to bring about macro-solutions that lead to a more just or equitable society.

People in middle-class and upper-class communities also suffer from mental illness and struggle with the shame and stigma that comes from this experience in the United States. The mental suffering of persons in the owning class or professional classes can also relate to contextual and autobiographical factors such as personal trauma. Persons in these class positions who suffer from mental distress continue to contribute, through discourse and meaning making, to the wider cultural world, and their voice, artistic contributions, and dignity must be honored. Pressures of class can attend persons who suffer with emotional distress in the upper echelons of society, so that they are burdened with added shame for transgressing their class norms.[17]

There is certainly a broader lens through which to view the impact of neoliberalism, even though this has not been this book's primary aim. Globalization indicates that working-class mental distress has been exported abroad. One factory worker at a hard disk manufacturer in Hunan Province, China, stated that she saw seven of her coworkers "going crazy at work," since they could not tolerate the constant threats and belittlement they experienced as a result of being in the working-class position in a Chinese factory.[18] Grappling with these other aspect of neoliberal globalism is beyond the scope of this project, yet it is important to note that neoliberalism has a global reach: The incitement to consume often means that others are consumed in the process.

In the end some may have wondered whether this focus on the causative contribution of economic oppression to mental illness was justified, asking if it implied that all mental illness could be stopped in an egalitarian society. The troubling implication here might be that mental illness was an identity to be dispensed with once the troubles of economic oppression were out of the way. This would be quite a different conclusion than the one reached by c/s/x activists who often reclaim aspects of their experience as a source of wisdom. Working on the frontiers of claiming their own truth and identity and claiming insight and creativity, many consider themselves in touch with a wider realm of truth than most of us.

Social aspects of emotional distress have been underemphasized in the United States, where it is less likely that differences will be tolerated. There is evidence that more egalitarian and communal societies have lower incidence of schizophrenia, much greater recovery rates, and in general a more positive attitude toward emotional distress.[19] The World Health Organization's epidemiology studies that have analyzed societies for several decades and indicate that rather than a universal biological reality, schizophrenia actually has a tremendously different course based on the cultural formation in the society where it is expressed.[20]

I argue that the extent of current economic oppression and the suffering caused by it can lead to shared solidarity, a feeling of understanding and an impetus to change limiting conditions. Concluding that this does not place a false distinction in the middle of mental suffering caused by economic factors and those caused by genetic or biological factors, but rather that it shows the much broader reach of emotional distress and how many more persons can respond to it and alleviate it.

Because of this book's focus, there has not been room to adequately address the concerns of families who care for persons with mental illness, although in an era of deinstitutionalization, the physical and financial pressures on them are quite substantial. There are important books that begin to do so, critiquing the state of mental health care in this nation and offering alternatives.[21]

Alternative Anthropologies to Neoliberalism

There are several ways that we can use an analysis of neoliberalism to challenge the psychotherapeutic approach to the human being with a more complex image of the person. While direct-to-consumer advertising might have attempted to persuade us that our happiness lies with what kind of drugs we can consume, we can challenge these outmoded notions of therapeutically produced happiness and ask about other values that are significant to us as people: grounded joy, deep connection, justice-based relationships, and shared access to valued goods. We are not empty because we lack pharmaceutical drugs, but our emptiness may be related to the cultural and social circumstances in which we live. Instead of attention or anxiety disorders, our primary problem may be compassion and justice disorders, the dulling of feeling and a lack of ability to see and respond to each other's needs.[22]

Ministerial authority can offer up a different image of the human being. At the same time, we can challenge the image of success given to us by a society oriented toward producing and consuming, offering instead images of shared solidarity as our role models for the good life. Religious leaders and counselors often offer implicit signs of who are their role models. In their speeches, prayers, and in the décor in their offices, they reveal who they look up to and venerate. Considering those important pioneers of religious communities such as Abraham Joshua Heschel, Dorothy Day, Martin Luther King, Jr., and César Chávez, persons whose faith inspired the changes that they wished to see, offers a notion of "presence" rooted in religious identity that revises stereotypes about worth and success. The lives of these leaders seem to indicate that personal success was indivisible from the social good and that neither of these could be separated from the worship of the Holy.

When we explore themes of mental illness and its inverse, mental health, we are always lifting up a mirror to society.[23] Doing this by suggesting what it is normative, we grapple with the fact that each opportunity to provide care and counsel is an exercise in language in which we use discourse. When we use this discourse we implicitly lift up certain visions of the good life even as we encourage persons to grow, to become healthy, to worship God, and to connect with one another.[24]

The people we counsel do not have an imbalance in their heads, they live in a society that is extremely unbalanced and that has largely lost track of what is good for itself and for one another. Stating it in this way, I do not presume that there was a golden age we could return to, but rather that we have silenced some significant calls for prophetic justice, rooted in faith, that used to be a significant part of religious life together in society. Reclaiming these calls for justice means offering a theological anthropology that challenges that notion of untrammeled greed and envy at the heart of neoliberal philosophy.[25] Believing in this deeper meaning for persons' lives means revising a pharmaceutical logic that suggests that people are empty until they are filled by certain compounds or substances.

Counter-Conducts in a Neoliberal Era

In the twenty-first century we also need more religious communities that exercise the counter-conducts on each other's behalf. These are communities that are characterized by solidarity in which the concerns that each other face become a central interest, lifted up in prayer and addressed in direct human conduct.

Ministers often feel that the care of the mentally ill is beyond their capacities, but they are frequently sought as front-line responders to mental distress. Grappling with the pain that comes from emotional distress is often what clergy do as part of their role of travelling with persons across time. Ministers are sought to help interpret mental distress: "Am I crazy, pastor?" asks the parishioner who is juggling two jobs, taking care of small children, and caring for an elderly parent at the same time, all the while simply trying to pay the rent and keep utilities on.

After reading this book, ministers will have an interpretive lens with which to decouple the stress that comes from economic circumstances from biomedical notions of mental illness. In the biomedical model, if someone is depressed it is the universal disease process that comes to the fore and depression, as a fixed entity, will have a course in the brains and bodies of persons. Yet through the framework offered in this book, ministers come to see how mental illness is frequently an effect of macro-stress, the pileup of chronic trauma, and the breakdown of bonds of community.[26] To address these sources of distress, ministers must use religious supports, specifically the resources of community.

In certain instances ministers become people who are sought to help interpret the complex kinds of suffering described in this book.

This invitation constitutes a certain kind of relationship that I have called pastoral power. In this book I have argued that pastoral power consists of three interlocking realities: trust deriving from the amount of time a minster has travelled with a community, symbolic power that comes from ordination, as well as shared cultural or experiential heritage. Pastoral power is the interpretive authority that derives from these three sources.

In my argument in these pages I maintain that pastoral power is best used when it is geared toward community liberation. For example, if a minister uses her power to reinforce a limited view of the human being based on his own needs and anxieties, this is a misuse of pastoral power. Likewise, the misuse of pastoral power can be more subtle and insidious, deriving from the lack of mention of certain social factors in ministerial discourse.

This does not mean that pastors should neglect to refer to mental health counselors in their communities, especially those who share an expansive vision for the social causes of suffering, but simply that they should not see the struggle against emotional suffering as ending there. Once a person has had their negative and positive symptoms of schizophrenia mapped, or their suffering charted with a depression scale from one to five, and once they are treated with psychiatric medication for a time, they may have addressed some of the effects of the situation they are facing, but they may return to an unchanged social and cultural environment. This means that frontline mental health work has to include macro elements as well as micro ones.[27]

It also means that this care must primarily be about how the community responds to each other rather than simply how a privileged expert uses their authority to interpret the lives of their community. In the counter-conducts of pastoral power people engage with each other so that they experience several crucial realities: the direct presence of God and the confirmation of oneself as a person worthy of love and respect that comes from God's dialogue with the soul. Through the counter-conducts of pastoral power there is the community that takes each person's story seriously and seeks to respond to it as if it were their own, the asceticism that is willing to give up some things for the greater good, the Scripture that confirms the soul's relationship to God in community with the most destitute, and an eschatology that tells us that God's work will be completed in relationships of justice that do not deny the traumas of history.

The neoliberal era has foreshortened time by focusing specifically on profit accumulation and the rapid transfer of capital across national borders.[28] In this new economy the future is only seen through the light of money, which provides a significant end toward which society is geared. If there is something other than money, for example, if there is God, prayer, or the soul, then it is a significant challenge to a neoliberal mindset, turning the idols of the present age on their head. The significant respect accorded to someone who has money is thereby challenged by rerouting people to a new system of evaluation, one in which even if they are not wealthy and are in debt, they are inviolable centers of value and personhood, regardless of their capacities.

Counter-conducts put to work in a neoliberal economy can thus resist the pressure that people face to make themselves into entrepreneurs by selling themselves as a kind of product. By contrast, they can help persons experience how they are seen and known by God first of all rather than through the attributes of money or social class. This is one of the primary and scandalous facts about the church in a neoliberal era: it is not a social club and it is not directed toward the accumulation of profit. Rather, it is an institution open to all and geared toward the glorification of God in the world. With this purpose in mind, worship, prayer, pastoral care, and religious education, are all sacred tasks that have no monetary value. Indeed, they challenge the monetization of the human being that is so much in vogue in the new economy.

What has to be transformed in religious communities for these counter-conducts to be effective is a set of interlocking taboos. At one Protestant congregation during the time of prayers, people often raise their hands and ask for physical illnesses to be cured. Rarely do people talk about emotional distress, and even more rarely about financial distress, namely the conditions of labor for those in the working class. From this vantage point, certain topics are being selected for religious concern and mobilization while others are left to the side.

By contrast, one minister explicitly links economic suffering with mental distress in his prayer time, lifting up all of those who "struggle to survive" in a new economy and felt "discouragement and fatigue" as a result. When sharing a story in the sermon the following week about someone in a working-class position who felt discouragement after repeated job loss, the minister said, "And that's our story as well isn't it? There's a lot of suffering in this community right now, and it isn't just one person's fault." Talking this way about the economy from the pulpit, the minister broadened the reach of the counter-conducts of pastoral power, allowing that which had been a taboo subject to be spoken publicly in a community

Reframing Authorities in Mental Health Care

Some have argued that ministers in a variety of settings need to get advanced training in counseling to help the people in their communities cope. This may be true in some instances. At the same time, ministers can also educate themselves from different sources, from the voices of c/s/x advocates in their own communities, many of whom address intersectional oppression in their advocacy for persons struggling with mental distress. I argue here that ministers should be oriented away from the professional experts in the psy-disciplines for authoritative witness to the experience of mental distress and shift their perspective toward the narratives of survivors, consumers, and ex-patients who have defined their own journeys of faith and life, hope and struggle. The best way to achieve solidarity is to allow voice to emerge.

Part of becoming thoughtful ministers to persons with mental distress is to listen to their own narratives rather than dismissing them because of mentalism. This is a central point that has emerged throughout the text, that by foregrounding the perspectives of persons struggling with mental health issues, clergy and other caregivers can hear about the concerns faced by persons in their communities and how they wish to have them addressed.

Frequently these concerns are not so much voices or hallucinations as they are housing, transportation, appropriate work, and unconditional friendship. Asking people about their own experience and how they understand it, including their material needs, brings the testimony of persons who have been in the mental health system to the foreground. Ministers should not be afraid to talk with persons about their hospitalizations or their feelings about medication, fraught issues that ministers often think exist beyond the scope of their practice. Yet for c/s/x activists in their community, these aspects of daily life are an arena of contestation and control in which complex images of the human being as embodied, created in the image of God, and worthy of dignity, come to the fore.

When a minister listens in community to the concerns of c/s/x activists, they become more likely to advocate around intersectional rights for them, such as good quality housing in a gentrified neighborhood, or the rights of a halfway house to remain in a community despite the not-in-my-backyard phenomenon.[29] Likewise, ministers can learn how to help persons prepare psychiatric advanced directives and negotiate with family and mental health providers to have these directives honored.[30] Given the discussion of deinstitutionalization in chapter 2, at times it is necessary for ministers to advocate for better and more widespread mental health care community services, including therapy as well as medication, in areas where mental health care is nonexistent.[31] Ministers can also become part of the boards of commissions that oversee psychiatric hospitals, visiting patients, and running religious services, but also overseeing the hospital to prevent abuses and to make certain that people are treated with dignity.

Coming alongside persons who have experienced emotional suffering thus means dealing with the fear of difference, of feeling over one's head, along with the perception that there is someone else more qualified than one's self to have conversations about mental illness. Reading materials written by survivors who talk about their own experience (many publications from the MIND organization in the United Kingdom meet this category) can reframe the authority base from which ministers help their parishioners.[32] Publications written by recovery organizations highlight people's own efforts to cope with mental illness symptoms. When ministers familiarize themselves with c/s/x based literature they balance professional expert perspectives with first-person stories about coping, stigma, oppression, managing unnecessary shame, objectification, and reentering community. Becoming versed in this literature, a minister might not simply refer a parishioner, but ask, "How have you found yourself coping during an especially tough time? Is there anything that you've learned to do that really helps?"

Of course, as one c/s/x activist claimed, what we are all hoping for is "a drug to cure the world of capitalism," but until we come up with that magic pill we will have to find a way to lessen its effects.[33] One of the ways to do this is through concerted efforts to honor and respect those who are less visible in our religious communities. This means speaking to them, hearing what they care about, and learning how they cope with their lives. How they cope with their struggles often provides insights for us into how we can cope with our own.

Oriented around the claims of mental health users rather than the official claims of persons who work in disciplines that regulate patients, ministers can hear different claims and evaluate knowledge from a different point of view. When this results in an orientation toward actively helping the person in their midst cope with and change the circumstances of their lives, rather than simply finding a professional to prescribe medications to them, ministers will move closer to being actual "partners" to the testimony of c/s/x survivors. Sometimes becoming partners means finding access to valued resources or networking for community support, and at other times it simply means getting out of the way of activists so that they can set their own agenda.

An Integrative Vision for Pastoral Power • 199

At a church where I was a parishioner I cohosted a conference on mental illness titled "People Are Not Problems to Be Solved, but Mysteries to Be Lived." The event was cohosted by a c/s/x activist who became hospitalized right before the event was scheduled to occur. On the day of the event, I met with one other person who attended the conference and later went to visit the c/s/x activist in the psychiatric hospital. While I had prepared for a presentation of the ideas in this book, the fact that my cohost had been hospitalized reframed the entire conversation. We began to talk, not in generalities, but about the specific c/s/x activist and the community support that he needed at the time. In this sense, the church was there in the midst of the everyday experience of communion with persons who had been diagnosed because of emotional distress.

C/S/X Activism: Resurrecting Silenced Stories

It is crucial that we revise our narratives about mental health and mental illness to foreground the stories of dignity and courage rather than emphasizing pathology. A man was picked up on the beach in Galveston Bay, Texas, and brought into the psychiatric hospital for evaluation, where it was discovered that he was a patient who had stayed at several other psychiatric hospitals. "He claimed to have graduated from Michigan State University... and also to have been the 'original integration leader in Texas.'" At this the psychiatrists scoffed, but he stated that he only had one desire left, namely, "to write his life story."[34] This story became the basis for the book, *No Color Is My Kind: The Life of Eldrewery Stearns and the Integration of Houston,* written by Thomas Cole.

In 1959 the Houston police picked up Stearns with the pretext of a malfunctioning taillight, and, once they discovered he had a white woman's photo in his wallet he was taken into custody, tortured and beaten. As a result of this experience Stearns became oriented toward activism. Through his work at the YMCA he became a leader in the integration movement. Incidentally, the integration of Houston happened during a media blackout imposed by the city authorities so that the world would not see what occurred there.

Cole described Stearns' courage and ingenuity, and closes the book by diagnosing him with a mental illness:

> By now, I hope readers will have some appreciation for Eldrewery Stearns as a fellow human being, as a unique and flawed historical figure. With great sadness—and against his vehement objections—I summarize in the following pages what I have learned about manic-depressive illness and what I believe is its place in his life story.[35]

Cole goes on to draw a picture of Stearns as exuding "charm," yet also having mood swings and drinking heavily and in doing so fits his story into a broader psychiatric frame.[36] Cole attempted to have Stearns treated by several psychiatrist friends by inviting them to come to his office to talk with Stearns.

Let me clarify: we can thank Cole for attending to Stearns' story even as we challenge the assumptions of the clinical frame with which he surrounds it. Although Stearns longs to have his story told, it also seems that he wishes to be remembered for his courage, his community activism, his trauma at the hands of white officers, and his resistance to this trauma. Unfortunately, the clinical frame revises some of these concrete particulars of Stearns' story.

In effect, Cole tells the world that Stearns is a mental patient despite his objections. It is not clear that this *telling of his story on his behalf*, describing to the world who he was *as* bipolar, was in Stearns' best interest. This description of Stearns as someone diagnosed with a mental illness displays the enormous power of the author.

Nevertheless, from this story, and from the documentary Cole made based on Stearns' life, one has a picture of a narrative that has escaped even the clinical frame assigned to it, showing the ingenuity involved in community organizing and the passion for the truth that impelled him. This was ultimately the passion of faith, conceived in the broadest sense.

Stearns insisted on his own self-definition in text and film[37] and resisted the all-encompassing nature of the mental diagnosis given to him. In some sense his story is a counter-witness to the privilege of those who would insist on writing about it.

In a now famous passage, Foucault maintains that there could be an "insurrection of subjugated knowledges... blocs of historical knowledge which were present but disguised within the body of functionalist and systematizing theory and which criticism—which obviously draws on scholarship—has been able to reveal."[38] As such, in the life of anyone given a diagnosis of mental illness, there are counter-narratives and stories that contradict this broader frame: these stories can be used as the fodder for new social movements.

Foucault indicates that resistance may be hiding in plain sight. I argue that we lack the interpretive lenses with which to understand this resistance because of the influence of psychiatric discourse. The insurrection of subjugated knowledge in the case means exploring the way that mental illness came to function as a primary identity marker, rather than categories of social and cultural oppression, activism or religious membership.

Yet another change occurs that is even more profound than this consciousness-raising activity. Ministers and pastoral counselors begin to witness their own entailment in these stories and thus move from being a supposedly objective, detached observer to being a "partner." This partnership requires them to act, perhaps by becoming part of a board that supports mental health users or visits local psychiatric hospitals or prisons in order to document the treatment of mental patients.[39] As Stearns' story indicates, persons who have been diagnosed with mental illness can organize for social change around a variety of identities. A key factor in this organization needs to be economic, since studies have indicated that persons with higher incomes tend to benefit more from mental health users activism.[40]

Conclusion

In writing this book I have sought to unsettle our taken-for-granted notions of mental health and health care and argued that socio-structural concerns must be in the foreground as we attempt to address mental distress. Of course, the problems described in these pages are multidirectional and multifaceted, so that a single solution to them is going to ring hollow. Likewise, simply understanding a new narrative is not adequate unless there is action to relieve the suffering that is present in our new economy.

Hoping for a rapprochement between quite different fields of discourse—social class within a community organizing framework and c/s/x activism in the psychological world, I have shown how two disparate problems overlap significantly in our time. This seems to be an underappreciated intersection in modern American culture.

I have used examples throughout the book that have linked the micro-social and macro-social world, although because of my discipline in pastoral care and counseling, my work on the micro-world may have seemed more nuanced and complex. This is simply a statement of further work that needs to be done.

Many of the recent gains in the labor movement, such as increasing the base pay for workers at some of the nation's largest retail chains, are likely to have positive psychosocial impacts on the mental health in our communities. When this happens, we can build on these gains and see the gains of community organizing and labor as contributing directly to the solutions that pastoral care has been hoping to address.[41] While pastoral caregivers may wish to see healthier families and communities, one of the primary ways to approach this change is through economic rights organizing.

At the same time, there is a role for individual care, for meeting vulnerable persons where they are and helping them interpret their lives, especially confirming to them that the widespread economic suffering of our neoliberal era is not their personal fault or a responsibility that should be placed on their shoulders. Even as ministers and counselors engage in this role, I hope to educate them into a broader macro-perspective, since I sense that what has traditionally been termed ministerial and therapeutic "burnout" is actually something related to the loss of power that comes from repeatedly addressing social concerns at a micro-level. By broadening out their advocacy, as Christina did in chapter 4, ministers can see progress in social change and thus directly contribute to alleviating the suffering that they would have otherwise seen in pastoral care.

Through a macro-and-micro focus, ministers can work for the good of society by acting globally while thinking locally, using the tools described in this book such as the counter-conducts of pastoral power and the inquiries about social class. In the process, ministers will of course need to take care of themselves, since the macro-processes that they are attempting to transform will not be resolved overnight. This helpful point of view transcends the notion of individual focus so often involved in pastoral care, a focus that actually contributes to the suffering of both the caregiver and the client. The appreciation of the long-term social changes sought through pastoral care and counseling leads us to consider the prayer written by Fr. Ken Untener when he worked in inner city Detroit:

> We cannot do everything, and there is a sense of liberation in that. This enables us to do something, and to do it very well...we are ministers, not messiahs. We are prophets of a future not our own.[42]

Notes

Introduction

1. William Avison, Jane D. McLeod, and Bernice A. Pescosolido, *Mental Health, Social Mirror* (New York: Springer Science & Business Media, 2007).
2. Jake Ryan and Charles Sackrey, *Strangers in Paradise: Academics from the Working Class*. 2nd ed. (Lanham, MD: University Press of America, 1995).
3. Carles Muntaner et al., "Socioeconomic Position and Major Mental Disorders," *Epidemiologic Reviews* 26, no. 1 (July 1, 2004): 53.
4. Carl I. Cohen and Sami Timimi, *Liberatory Psychiatry: Philosophy, Politics, and Mental Health* (Cambridge, UK; New York: Cambridge University Press, 2008).
5. Ibid.; Vijaya Murali and Femi Oyebode, "Poverty, Social Inequality and Mental Health," *Advances in Psychiatric Treatment* 10, no. 3 (May 1, 2004): 216.
6. Stephen M. Petterson and Alison Burke Albers, "Effects of Poverty and Maternal Depression on Early Child Development," *Child Development* 72, no. 6 (2001): 1794; Susan H. Spence et al., "Maternal Anxiety and Depression, Poverty and Marital Relationship Factors during Early Childhood as Predictors of Anxiety and Depressive Symptoms in Adolescence," *Journal of Child Psychology and Psychiatry* 43, no. 4 (2002): 457.
7. David Harvey, *A Brief History of Neoliberalism* (Oxford; New York: Oxford University Press, 2005): 2. Neoliberalism must be distinguished from liberal politics since its primary focus is "freeing" markets to operate independently. It can likewise be distinguished from neoconservativism that has a moralistic tone but similar political consequences.
8. Nick Couldry, *Why Voice Matters: Culture and Politics After Neoliberalism* (London: Sage, 2010).
9. Harvey Cox, "The Market as God," *The Atlantic*, March 1999.
10. Harvey, *A Brief History of Neoliberalism*.
11. Rogers-Vaughn, "Blessed Are Those Who Mourn: Depression as Political Resistance," *Pastoral Psychology* (2013): 506.

12. Ann Cvetkovich, *Depression: A Public Feeling* (Durham, NC; London: Duke University Press, 2012): 5.
13. Rogers-Vaughn, "Blessed Are Those Who Mourn." 1–20.
14. Rogers-Vaughn cites queer feminist Ann Cvetkovich's work *Depression: A Public Feeling*, as one instance of this resistance in the "public feelings" project that situates depression as a response to cultural and social circumstances against which typical organizing has been ineffective. Cvetkovich cites queer theorists such as Douglas Crimp, Heather Love, and Jonathan Flatley who are linking emotional distress with rage and the capacity to resist and transform society.
15. Richard U'Ren, *Social Perspective: The Missing Element in Mental Health Practice* (Toronto; Buffalo: University of Toronto Press, Scholarly Publishing Division, 2011): 50.
16. Nikolas S. Rose, *Governing the Soul: The Shaping of the Private Self* (London; New York: Routledge, 1990): p. x.
17. Stephen Pattison, *Pastoral Care and Liberation* (Cambridge; New York: Cambridge University Press, 1994).
18. Adrienne S. Chambon, Allan Irving, and Laura Epstein, *Reading Foucault for Social Work* (New York: Columbia University Press, 1999). In his chapter in this text, Ken Moffatt describes how social workers engage in surveillance of welfare recipients through practices of forms, files, and panopticon-like office spaces, but how social workers sometimes collaborate with clients to resist this imposition of power by suggesting forms of resistance, p. 230.
19. In teaching about this subject, I had a student who had observed this phenomenon while working at a wealthy hospital.
20. Rose, *Governing the Soul*, p. 192.
21. Adrienne S. Chambon, Allan Irving, and Laura Epstein, *Reading Foucault for Social Work* (NewYork: Columbia University Press).
22. Patricia A. Joyce, "The Case Conference as Social Ritual Constructing a Mother of a Sexually Abused Child," *Qualitative Social Work* 4, no. 2 (June 1, 2005): 157–173.
23. Ken Moffatt, "Surveillance and Government of the Welfare Recipient," in *Reading Foucault for Social Work* (New York: Columbia University Press, 1999): 219–245.
24. David Smail, *Power, Interest and Psychology* (Ross-on-Wye: PCCS Books, 2013): 23.
25. Allan V. Horwitz, *The Loss of Sadness: How Psychiatry Transformed Normal Sorrow into Depressive Disorder* (Oxford; New York: Oxford University Press, 2007).
26. Marcia Angell, "Excess in the Pharmaceutical Industry," *CMAJ: Canadian Medical Association Journal* 171, no. 12 (December 7, 2004): 1451–1453.
27. Smail, *Power, Interest and Psychology*, iii.
28. Ibid., iv.

29. Ibid., 35.
30. Ibid., 32.
31. Cvetkovich, *Depression*, 5.
32. Hooks, *Where We Stand*.
33. Ibid., 28.
34. Ibid., 42.
35. Rogers-Vaughn, "Blessed Are Those Who Mourn."
36. Cushman, *Constructing The Self, Constructing America*, 185.
37. Philip Cushman, *Constructing the Self, Constructing America: A Cultural History of Psychotherapy* (Cambridge, MA: Da Capo Press, 1996): 185.
38. McClure, *Moving Beyond Individualism in Pastoral Care and Counseling*.
39. Liran Razinsky, *Freud, Psychoanalysis and Death* (Cambridge, UK: Cambridge University Press, 2013): 117.
40. Matt Bloom, "Are the Poor Happier? Perspectives from Business Management," in *The Preferential Option for the Poor Beyond Theology* (Notre Dame, IN: University of Notre Dame Press, 2014): 69–82.
41. Axel Honneth and Fraser, *Redistribution or Recognition? A Political-Philosophical Exchange* (London and New York: Verso, 2003).
42. Heather E. Bullock, "Justifying Inequality: A Social Psychological Analysis of Beliefs about Poverty and the Poor," in *The Colors of Poverty: Why Racial and Ethnic Disparities Persist* (New York: Sage Publications, 2008).
43. Honneth and Fraser, *Redistribution or Recognition?*
44. Chris Allen, "The Poverty of Death: Social Class, Urban Deprivation, and the Criminological Consequences of Sequestration of Death," *Mortality* 12, no. 1 (2007): 79–93. Even in cases such as bereavement, social class impacts how common psychological distress is experienced and the resources that one has to cope with it.
45. Deborah Marks, *Disability: Controversial Debates and Psychosocial Perspectives* (London; New York: Routledge, 1999): p. 18.
46. Patricia B. Nemec, LeRoy Spaniol and Arthur E. Dell Orto, "Psychiatric Rehabilitation Education," *Rehabilitation Education* 15, no. 2 (n.d.): 116.
47. Donal Dorr, *Option for the Poor and for the Earth: Catholic Social Teaching*, 20th anniversary ed. (Maryknoll, NY: Orbis Books, 2012): p. 174.
48. Linda Joy Morrison, *Talking Back to Psychiatry: The Psychiatric Consumer/Survivor/Ex-Patient Movement* (New York: Routledge, 2005).
49. Ronald Bassman, "Overcoming the Impossible," http://www.psychologytoday.com/articles/200101/overcoming-the-impossible, January 1, 2001.
50. Ibid.
51. Mark Creswell, "Psychiatric 'Survivors' and Testimonies of Self-Harm," *Social Science and Medicine*, 61 (2005): 1670.
52. E. S. J. Rogers et al., "A Consumer-Constructed Scale to Measure Empowerment among Users of Mental Health Services," *Psychiatric Services (Washington, D.C.)* 48, no. 8 (August 1997): 1042–1047.
53. Ibid.

54. Vicente Navarro et al., *Political and Economic Determinants of Population Health and Well-Being: Controversies and Developments* (Amityville, NY: Baywood 2004).
55. Michel Foucault, *Security, Territory, Population: Lectures at the Collège de France 1977–1978*. 1st ed. (New York: Picador, 2009).
56. Rogers et al., "A Consumer-Constructed Scale."

1 Social Class and Mental Illness in a Neoliberal Era

1. *Two American Families*. Frontline. Documentary film. Accessed February 4, 2015. http://www.pbs.org/wgbh/pages/frontline/two-american-families/.
2. Ibid.
3. Robert Putnam, *Our Kids: The American Dream in Crisis* (New York: Simon and Schuster, 2015).
4. Joerg Rieger, *No Rising Tide: Theology, Economics, and the Future* (Minneapolis, MN: Fortress Press, 2009).
5. This is also a concern for worker's rights since few overseas factories have worker protections.
6. Prabhat Patnaik, *Retreat to Unfreedom*: Essays on the Emerging World Order (New Delhi: Tulika, 2003).
7. Rogers-Vaughn, "Blessed Are Those Who Mourn: Depression as Political Resistance," *Pastoral Psychology* (2013): 1–20.
8. Michael White, *Narratives of Therapists' Lives* (Adelaide, South Australia: Dulwich Centre Publications, 1997): 57.
9. Michel Foucault, *The History of Sexuality* (New York: Vintage Books, 1990): 142.
10. Carles Muntaner et al., "Class Exploitation and Psychiatric Disorders: From Status Syndrome to Capitalist Syndrome," in *Liberatory Psychiatry* (Cambridge, UK; New York: Cambridge University Press, 2008): 132.
11. Carles Muntaner et al., "Socioeconomic Position and Major Mental Disorders," *Epidemiologic Reviews* 26, no. 1 (2004): 53–62.
12. V. Lorant et al., "Socioeconomic Inequalities in Depression: A Meta-Analysis," *American Journal of Epidemiology* 157, no. 2 (2003): 98–112.
13. William W. Eaton et al., "Socioeconomic Status and Depressive Syndrome: The Role of Inter- and Intra-Generational Mobility, Government Assistance, and Work Environment," *Journal of Health and Social Behavior* 42, no. 3 (September 1, 2001): 277–294.
14. Muntaner et al., "Class Exploitation and Psychiatric Disorders," 133.
15. R. M. Díaz et al., "The Impact of Homophobia, Poverty, and Racism on the Mental Health of Gay and Bisexual Latino Men: Findings from 3 US Cities," *American Journal of Public Health* 91, no. 6 (2001): 927.
16. Muntaner et al., "Class Exploitation and Psychiatric Disorders, 135.
17. S. Weich and G. Lewis, "Material Standard of Living, Social Class, and the Prevalence of the Common Mental Disorders in Great Britain," *Journal of Epidemiology and Community Health* 52, no. 1 (January 1, 1998): 11.

18. Ibid.
19. Lorant et al., "Socioeconomic Inequalities in Depression."
20. Muntaner et al., "Class Exploitation and Psychiatric Disorders."
21. Muntaner et al., "Socioeconomic Position and Major Mental Disorders."
22. Philip Thomas, *The Dialectics of Schizophrenia* (London; New York: Free Association Books, 1997).
23. Bruce P., *Adversity, Stress, and Psychopathology* (New York: Oxford University Press, 1998): 402.
24. Ibid., 404–405.
25. Connie R. Wanberg, "The Individual Experience of Unemployment," *Annual Review of Psychology* 63, no. 1 (2012): 370.
26. Gordon E. O'Brien, *Psychology of Work and Unemployment*, vol. xiii, Wiley Series in Psychology and Productivity at Work (Oxford, England: John Wiley & Sons, 1986).
27. "Bureau of Labor Statistics Data." Accessed January 12, 2015. http://data.bls.gov/timeseries/LNU04000000?years_option=all_years&periods_option=specific_periods&periods=Annual+Data.
28. Karsten I. Paul and Klaus Moser, "Unemployment Impairs Mental Health: Meta-Analyses," *Journal of Vocational Behavior* 74, no. 3 (2009): 264–282.
29. Ibid., 372.
30. "The Best—and Worst—Places to Lose Your Job." *BBC Capital*. Accessed March 10, 2015. http://www.bbc.com/capital/story/20141217-the-worst-countries-for-sacking.
31. Connie R. Wanberg, "The Individual Experience of Unemployment," *Annual Review of Psychology* 63, no. 1 (2012): 369–396.
32. Yiannis Gabriel, David E. Gray, and Harshita Goregaokar, "Temporary Derailment or the End of the Line? Managers Coping with Unemployment at 50," *Organization Studies* 31, no. 12 (December 1, 2010): 1687–1712.
33. Richard H. Price, Jin Nam Choi, and Amiram D. Vinokur, "Links in the Chain of Adversity Following Job Loss: How Financial Strain and Loss of Personal Control Lead to Depression, Impaired Functioning, and Poor Health," *Journal of Occupational Health Psychology* 7, no. 4 (October 2002): 302–312.
34. Ulrich A. Reininghaus et al., "Unemployment, Social Isolation, Achievement–Expectation Mismatch and Psychosis: Findings from the ÆSOP Study," *Social Psychiatry and Psychiatric Epidemiology* 43, no. 9 (September 1, 2008): 743–751.
35. Noa Sadeh and Rachel Karniol, "The Sense of Self-Continuity as a Resource in Adaptive Coping with Job Loss," *Journal of Vocational Behavior* 80, no. 1 (February 2012): 93–99.
36. David L. Blustein, Saliha Kozan, and Alice Connors-Kellgren, "Unemployment and Underemployment: A Narrative Analysis about Loss," *Journal of Vocational Behavior* 82, no. 3 (June 2013): 259.

37. Steven Stack and Ira Wasserman, "Economic Strain and Suicide Risk: A Qualitative Analysis," *Suicide and Life-Threatening Behavior* 37, no. 1 (2007): 103–112.
38. Ibid.
39. Doug Henwood, "American Dream: It's Not Working." *Christianity and Crisis* 52, no. 9 (June 8, 1992): 195–197.
40. Gérard Duménil, *The Crisis of Neoliberalism* (Cambridge, MA: Harvard University Press, 2013).
41. Ibid., 150.
42. Eva Selenko and Bernad Batinic, "Beyond Debt: A Moderator Analysis of the Relationship between Perceived Financial Strain and Mental Health," *Social Science & Medicine* 73, no. 12 (December 2011): 1725–1732.
43. ElinaTurunen and Heikki Hiilamo, "Health Effects of Indebtedness: A Systematic Review," *BMC Public Health* 14, no. 1 (May 22, 2014): 1.
44. Patricia Drentea and John R. Reynolds, "Neither a Borrower Nor a Lender Be," *Journal of Aging and Health* 24, no. 4 (2012): 673–695.
45. H. Meltzer et al., "Personal Debt and Suicidal Ideation," *Psychological Medicine* 41, no. 4 (April 2011): 771–778.
46. Turunen and Hiilamo, "Health Effects of Indebtedness."
47. Ibid., 4.
48. Sarah Bridges and Richard Disney, "Debt and Depression," *Journal of Health Economics* 29, no. 3 (May 2010): 388–403.
49. Turunen and Hiilamo, "Health Effects of Indebtedness," 6.
50. S. Hatcher, "Debt and Deliberate Self-Poisoning," *The British Journal of Psychiatry* 164, no. 1 (January 1, 1994): 111–114.
51. Melinda E. Cooper, *Life As Surplus: Biotechnology and Capitalism in the Neoliberal Era*, 1st ed. (Seattle, WA: University of Washington Press, 2008).
52. Jerry Mander, *The Capitalism Papers: Fatal Flaws of an Obsolete System* (Berkeley, CA: Counterpoint, 2013).
53. Karen Weise, "Bundled Mortgages Pose Problems for Housing Program," *ProPublica*. Accessed January 13, 2015. http://www.propublica.org/article/making-home-affordable-loan-modifications-denied-806.
54. Turunen and Hiilamo, "Health Effects of Indebtedness," 4.
55. Duménil, *The Crisis of Neoliberalism*, 151.
56. "2014 Year-End U.S. Foreclosure Market Report | Newsroom and Media Center." Accessed March 10, 2015. http://www.realtytrac.com/news/foreclosure-trends/1-1-million-u-s-properties-with-foreclosure-filings-in-2014-down-18-percent-from-2013-to-lowest-level-since-2006/.
57. "Economic Scarring: The Long-Term Impacts of the Recession," *Economic Policy Institute*. Accessed March 10, 2015.
58. K. A. McLaughlin et al., "Home Foreclosure and Risk of Psychiatric Morbidity during the Recent Financial Crisis," *Psychological Medicine* 42, no. 7 (July 2012): 1441–1448.

59. Jason N. Houle, "Mental Health in the Foreclosure Crisis," *Social Science & Medicine* 118 (October 2014): 3.
60. Ibid., 4.
61. John Gathergood, "Debt and Depression: Causal Links and Social Norm Effects," *The Economic Journal* 122, no. 563 (2012): 1094–1114.
62. Price, Choi, and Vinokur, "Links in the Chain of Adversity Following Job Loss."
63. Karsten I. Paul and Klaus Moser, "Unemployment Impairs Mental Health: Meta-Analyses," *Journal of Vocational Behavior* 74, no. 3 (2009): 264–282.
64. Carl Walker, *Depression and Globalization: The Politics of Mental Health in the 21st Century* (New York: Springer, 2008):140.
65. Richard U'Ren, *Social Perspective: The Missing Element in Mental Health Practice*, 1st ed. (Toronto; Buffalo, NY: University of Toronto Press, Scholarly Publishing Division, 2011).
66. George W. Brown and Patricia M. Moran, "Single Mothers, Poverty and Depression," *Psychological Medicine* 27, no. 1 (January 1997): 21–33.
67. Muntaner et al., "Class Exploitation and Psychiatric Disorders," 134.
68. Steve Lerner, *Sacrifice Zones: The Front Lines of Toxic Chemical Exposure in the United States* (Cambridge, MA: MIT Press, 2010).
69. John W. Lynch, George A. Kaplan, and Sarah J. Shema, "Cumulative Impact of Sustained Economic Hardship on Physical, Cognitive, Psychological, and Social Functioning," *New England Journal of Medicine* 337, no. 26 (December 25, 1997): 1894.
70. U'Ren, *Social Perspective*.
71. Weich and Lewis, "Material Standard of Living, Social Class, and the Prevalence of the Common Mental Disorders in Great Britain," 11.
72. Perrucci, *The New Class Society*, 32.
73. Henwood, "American Dream."
74. Rieger, *No Rising Tide*, 40.
75. Robert Perrucci, *The New Class Society: Goodbye American Dream?* 3rd ed. (Lanham, MD: Rowman & Littlefield Publishers, 2007).
76. Rieger, *No Rising Tide*, 41.
77. Center for Community Economic Development, "Closing the Racial Wealth Gap."
78. "USDA Economic Research Service—Geography of Poverty." Accessed February 21, 2015. http://www.ers.usda.gov/topics/rural-economy-population/rural-poverty-well-being/geography-of-poverty.aspx.
79. Duménil, *The Crisis of Neoliberalism*.
80. Perrucci, *The New Class Society*.
81. Ibid.
82. Harvey, *A Brief History of Neoliberalism*.
83. Walker, *Depression and Globalization*,68.
84. Ibid., 103.

85. B. J. Brown and Sally Baker, *Responsible Citizens: Individuals, Health and Policy under Neoliberalism* (New York: Anthem Press, 2013).
86. Erik Olin Wright, *Approaches to Class Analysis* (Cambridge, UK; New York: Cambridge University Press, 2005): 7.
87. Ibid., 24.
88. Asen, *Visions of Poverty: Welfare Policy and Political Imagination* (East Lansing, MI: MSU Press, 2012): 25.
89. Wright, *Approaches to Class Analysis*.
90. Carles Muntaner et al., "Social Class, Assets, Organizational Control and the Prevalence of Common Groups of Psychiatric Disorders," *Social Science & Medicine* 47, no. 12 (1998): 2043–2053.
91. Carles Muntaner et al., "Socioeconomic Position and Major Mental Disorders," *Epidemiologic Reviews* 26, no. 1 (2004): 53–62.
92. Carles Muntaner et al., "Class Relations and All-Cause Mortality: A Test of Wright's Social Class Scheme Using the Barcelona 2000 Health Interview Survey," *International Journal of Health Services: Planning, Administration, Evaluation* 41, no. 3 (2011): 431–458.
93. Ibid.
94. Wright, *Approaches to Class Analysis*, 22.
95. Steve Biko, *I Write What I Like: Selected Writings*, ed. Aelred Stubbs C.R. 1st ed. (Chicago: University of Chicago Press, 2002): ix.
96. Mikhail Aleksandrovich Bakunin, *Marxism, Freedom and the State* (MT: Kessinger Publishing, 2004).
97. Perrucci, *The New Class Society*, 29.
98. Erik Olin Wright, *Envisioning Real Utopias*, 1st ed. (London; New York: Verso, 2010): 286.
99. Christina Pantazis, David Gordon, and Ruth Levitas, *Poverty and Social Exclusion in Britain: The Millennium Survey*. Policy Press, 2006, 137.
100. US Census Bureau Public Information Office, "Nearly 1 in 5 People Have a Disability in the U.S., Census Bureau Reports – Miscellaneous – Newsroom – U.S. Census Bureau." Accessed March 10, 2015. https://www.census.gov/newsroom/releases/archives/miscellaneous/cb12-134.html.
101. Slorach, "Marxism and Disability." *International Socialism* 129.
102. Zygmunt Bauman, *Liquid Times* (Cambridge; MA: Polity Press): 70.
103. James I. Charlton, *Nothing about Us without Us: Disability Oppression and Empowerment* (Berkeley: University of California Press, 1998): 24.
104. Ibid.
105. Nev Jones and Robyn Brown, "The Absence of Psychiatric C/S/X Perspectives in Academic Discourse: Consequences and Implications," *Disability Studies Quarterly* 33, no. 1 (December 18, 2012).
106. Kimberle Crenshaw, "Mapping the Margins: Intersectionality, Identity Politics, and Violence against Women of Color," *Stanford Law Review* 43, no. 6 (July 1, 1991): 244.

107. Muntaner et al., "Class Exploitation and Psychiatric Disorders," 139.
108. George Monbiot, "Sick of This Market-Driven World? You Should Be," *The Guardian*, August 5, 2014.
109. Richard Sennett, *The Hidden Injuries of Class*, 1st ed. (New York: Knopf, 1972).
110. Heather E. Bullock, "Justifying Inequality: A Social Psychological Analysis of Beliefs about Poverty and the Poor," in *The Colors of Poverty: Why Racial and Ethnic Disparities Persist* (New York: Sage Publications, 2008): 53.
111. Rieger, *No Rising Tide*, 43.
112. Bullock, "Justifying Inequality."
113. Ibid., 55.
114. Ann Chih Lin and Harris, *The Colors of Poverty: Why Racial and Ethnic Disparities Persist* (New York: Russell Sage Foundation, 2008): 55.
115. Matthew O. Hunt, "Race/Ethnicity and Beliefs about Wealth and Poverty," *Social Science Quarterly* 85, no. 3 (September 2004): 841.
116. Oscar Lewis, "The Culture of Poverty," *Society* 35, no. 2 (1998): 7–9.
117. Herbert Gans, *The War against the Poor: The Underclass and Antipoverty Policy* (New York: Basic Books, 1996).
118. Alice O'Connor, *Poverty Knowledge: Social Science, Social Policy, and the Poor in Twentieth-Century U.S. History*, reprint ed. (Princeton, NJ: Princeton University Press, 2002).
119. Gavin Roger Jones, *American Hungers: The Problem of Poverty in U.S. Literature, 1840–1945* (Princeton, NJ: Princeton University Press, 2008).
120. Gunnar Myrdal, *Challenge to Affluence* (New York: Random House, 1963).
121. Gans, *The War against the Poor*, 36.
122. Ibid., 38.
123. Ibid., 41.
124. Ibid., 123.
125. Muntaner, Borrell, and Chung, "Class Relations, Economic Inequality and Mental Health," 136.
126. Ibid.
127. Ibid.
128. Ibid., 136.
129. Perrucci, *The New Class Society*.
130. Joerg Rieger, *Religion, Theology, and Class: Fresh Engagements after Long Silence* (New York: Palgrave Macmillan, 2013): 199.
131. Ibid., 200.
132. Theodore W. Allen and State University of New York at Stony Brook Center for Study of Working Class Life, *Class Struggle and the Origin of Racial Slavery: The Invention of the White Race* (Center for the Study of Working Class Life, Dept. of Economics, State University of New York, 2006).

133. Wright, *Envisioning Real Utopias*, 12.
134. Ibid., 4.
135. Ibid., 79.
136. Jung Mo Sung, "Greed, Desire and Theology," *The Ecumenical Review* 63, no. 3 (October 2011): 251.
137. "Two American Families."
138. Philip S. Wang, Patricia A. Berglund, and Ronald C. Kessler, "Patterns and Correlates of Contacting Clergy for Mental Disorders in the United States," *Health Services Research* 38, no. 2 (April 2003): 647–673.
139. Linda M. Chatters et al., "Use of Ministers for a Serious Personal Problem among African Americans: Findings from the National Survey of American Life," *The American Journal of Orthopsychiatry* 81, no. 1 (January 2011): 118–127.
140. Carroll A. Ali, *Survival & Liberation : Pastoral Theology in African American Context* (St. Louis, MO: Chalice Press, 1999).
141. "Bureau of Labor Statistics Data."
142. Jackson W. Carroll, *God's Potters: Pastoral Leadership and the Shaping of Congregations* (Grand Rapids, MI: Wm. B. Eerdmans Publishing Company, 2006).
143. "Bureau of Labor Statistics Data."
144. Carroll, *God's Potters*.
145. Ibid.
146. "Presbyterian Church (U.S.A.)—News & Announcements—Moonlighting Pastors and Postponed Health Care," April 8, 2014.
147. Sarah Brown, Karl Taylor, and Stephen Wheatley Price, "Debt and Distress: Evaluating the Psychological Cost of Credit," *Journal of Economic Psychology* 26, no. 5 (2005): 642–663.
148. Carroll, *God's Potters*, 93.
149. Ibid., 64.
150. Rogers-Vaughn, "Blessed Are Those Who Mourn."
151. Richard Gula, *Just Ministry: Professional Ethics for Pastoral Ministers*, (New York: Paulist Press, 2010): 30.
152. Erik Olin Wright, *Class Counts*: *Comparative Studies in Class Analysis* (Cambridge; New York: Paris: Cambridge University Press, 1996): 22.
153. Katherine Burgess, "Report: Church Giving Reaches Depression-Era Record Lows," *The Washington Post*, October 24, 2013.
154. Rieger, *No Rising Tide*.

2   Psychiatric Power and the Limits of Biomedical Diagnosis

1. "Part 1, How Mad Are You? 2008–2009, Horizon—BBC Two." *BBC*. Accessed February 6, 2015.
2. David L. Rosenhan, "On Being Sane in Insane Places," *Science: New Series* 179, no. 4070 (1973): 250–2050.

3. Ibid., 2052.
4. Ibid., 2053.
5. Ibid., 2052.
6. Eugen Bleuler, *Dementia Praecox; Or, The Group of Schizophrenias*. Monograph Series on Schizophrenia; No. 1 (New York, International Universities Press, 1950).
7. "The Pseudo-Patient Study, Mind Changers—BBC Radio 4." Accessed February 6, 2015.
8. Peter Conrad, *The Medicalization of Society: On the Transformation of Human Conditions into Treatable Disorders* (Baltimore: Johns Hopkins University Press, 2007).
9. Gary Greenberg, *Manufacturing Depression: The Secret History of a Modern Disease* (New York: Simon & Schuster, 2010).
10. Arthur Kleinman, *Rethinking Psychiatry : From Cultural Category to Personal Experience* (New York: London: Free Press; Collier Macmillan, 1991).
11. Ibid., 12.
12. Ibid., 117.
13. Thomas Philip and Patrick J. Bracken, *Postpsychiatry* (Oxford; New York: Oxford University Press, 2005).
14. David L. Rosenhan, "On Being Sane in Insane Places," *Science: New Series* 179, no. 4070 (1973): 179.
15. Michel Foucault, *Power/Knowledge: Selected Interviews and Other Writings, 1972–1977* (New York: Pantheon Books, 1980): 112.
16. Michel Foucault, *The History of Sexuality* (New York: Vintage Books, 1990): 28.
17. Ibid., 27.
18. Foucault, *Power/Knowledge*, 107.
19. Joffe-Walt, "Unfit for Work," National Public Radio: http://apps.npr.org/unfit-for-work/.
20. "CDC: Mental Disorders Rising in Children." Accessed February 6, 2015.
21. Ibid.
22. "QuickStats: Prevalence of Current Depression among Persons Aged ≥12 Years, by Age Group and Sex—United States, National Health and Nutrition Examination Survey, 2007–2010." Accessed February 6, 2015.
23. "CDC."
24. Conrad, *The Medicalization of Society*, 4.
25. Peter Conrad and Caitlin Slodden, "The Medicalization of Mental Disorder," in *Handbook of the Sociology of Mental Health*, 2nd ed. (New York: Springer, 2013): 61–73.
26. Hicks, "Reducing Disparities in the Use of Treatments for Depression and Other Mood Disorders."
27. Greenberg, *Manufacturing Depression*.

28. Ibid., 65.
29. Ibid., 70.
30. Dan G. Blazer, *The Age of Melancholy*: *"Major Depression" and Its Social Origin* (New York: Routledge, 2005): 50.
31. Greenberg, *Manufacturing Depression*, 69.
32. Ibid., 78.
33. David Healy, *The Antidepressant Era*, reprint ed. (Cambridge, MA: Harvard University Press, 1999).
34. Ibid., 27.
35. Healy, *The Antidepressant Era*.
36. Conrad, *The Medicalization of Society*.
37. Healy, *The Antidepressant Era*, 53.
38. Healy, *The Antidepressant Era*.
39. Geddes et al., "Selective Serotonin Reuptake Inhibitors (SSRIs) versus Other Antidepressants for Depression," in *The Cochrane Database of Systematic Reviews* (Hoboken, NJ: John Wiley & Sons, 1996).
40. Healy, *The Antidepressant Era*, 164.
41. Ibid., 109.
42. Ibid., 47.
43. Ibid., 160.
44. Angell, "Excess in the Pharmaceutical Industry," *CMAJ : Canadian Medical Association Journal* 171, no. 12 (December 7, 2004): 1451–1453.
45. Greenberg, *Manufacturing Depression*.
46. Geddes et al., "Selective Serotonin Reuptake Inhibitors (SSRIs) versus Other Antidepressants for Depression."
47. Ibid.
48. Healy, *The Antidepressant Era*, 212.
49. Healy, *The Antidepressant Era*.
50. Ibid., 227.
51. Ibid., 231.
52. Michael K. Steinberg, Joseph J Hobbs (Joseph John), and Kent Mathewson, *Dangerous Harvest*: *Drug Plants and the Transformation of Indigenous Landscapes* (New York: Oxford University Press, 2004).
53. Healy, *The Antidepressant Era*, 169.
54. Blazer, *The Age of Melancholy*, 8.
55. Gary Greenberg, *The Book of Woe, The DSM and the Unmaking of Psychiatry* (New York: Blue Rider Press, a member of Penguin Group USA Inc, 2013): 40.
56. Healy, *The Antidepressant Era*.
57. American Psychiatric Association, *Diagnostic and Statistical Manual of Mental Disorders* (DSM Library, American Psychiatric Association, 2013).
58. B. Rogers-Vaughn, "Blessed Are Those Who Mourn: Depression as Political Resistance," *Pastoral Psychology* (2013): 507.

59. Healy, *The Antidepressant Era*, 237.
60. Greenberg, *Manufacturing Depression*.
61. Blazer, *The Age of Melancholy*, 59.
62. Ibid., 64.
63. Frantz Fanon, *Black Skin, White Masks* (New York: Grove Press; Berkeley, CA, 2008): 165.
64. Ibid., 130.
65. Ibid., 73.
66. Mark S. Micale and Roy Porter, *Discovering the History of Psychiatry* (New York: Oxford University Press, 1994): 400.
67. Thomas Szasz, *The Myth of Mental Illness: Foundations of a Theory of Personal Conduct*, revised ed. (New York, Harper & Row, 1974): 61.
68. Ibid., 28.
69. Thomas Szasz, "Varieties of Psychiatric Criticism," *History of Psychiatry* 23, no. 3 (September 1, 2012): 355.
70. Erich Fromm, *The Sane Society* (New York: Fawcett Premier, 1955): 71.
71. Ibid., 111.
72. Ibid., 129.
73. Hyon-Uk Shin, *Vulnerability and Courage a Pastoral Theology of Poverty and the Alienated Self* (New York: Peter Lang, 2012).
74. Fromm, *The Sane Society*, 172.
75. Ibid., 211.
76. Blazer, *The Age of Melancholy*, 89.
77. Jonathan Metzl, *The Protest Psychosis: How Schizophrenia Became a Black Disease* (Boston: Beacon Press, 2009): 39.
78. Phyllis Chesler, *Women and Madness* (San Diego: Harcourt Brace Jovanovich, 1989).
79. Jennifer Rebecca Levison, "Elizabeth Parsons Ware Packard: An Advocate for Cultural, Religious, and Legal Change," *Alabama Law Review* 54 (2003, 2002): 985.
80. M. Loring and B. Powell, "Gender, Race and DSM-Iii: A Study of the Objectivity of Psychiatric Diagnostic Behavior," *Journal of Health and Social Behavior* 29, no. 1 (1988): 10.
81. Loring and Powell, "Gender, Race and DSM-Iii," 10.
82. Metzl, *The Protest Psychosis*, xv.
83. Ibid., xiv.
84. Ibid.
85. Ibid., 94.
86. Ibid., 117.
87. Vilma Santiago-Irizarry, *Medicalizing Ethnicity: The Construction of Latino Identity in a Psychiatric Setting* (Ithaca, NY: Cornell University Press, 2001): 67.
88. Ibid., 136.
89. Ibid., 133.

90. Ibid., 99.
91. Ibid., 42, 93.
92. Carrie Doehring, *The Practice of Pastoral Care: A Postmodern Approach* (Louisville, KY: Westminster John Knox Press, 2006).
    In the third chapter Carrie Doehring has a section on cultural competence, but then describes assessing "cultural liabilities" later in the book when she uses a series of charts and assessment strategies.
    John Patton, *Pastoral Care in Context: An Introduction to Pastoral Care* (Louisville, KY: Westminster/John Knox Press, 1993).
93. Nikolas S. Rose, *Governing the Soul: The Shaping of the Private Self* (London; New York: Routledge, 1990): xvii.
94. Loring and Powell, "Gender, Race and DSM-Iii," 9.
95. Metzl, *The Protest Psychosis*, 187.
96. Richard H. Lamb and Linda E. Weinberger, "Persons with Severe Mental Illness in Jails and Prisons," A Review," *Psychiatric Services* 49, no. 4 (April 1, 1998): 484.
97. Ibid.
98. Steven Raphael and Michael A. Stoll, *Why Are So Many Americans in Prison?* (New York: Russell Sage Foundation, 2013): 124.
99. Ibid., 152.
100. Ibid., 130.
101. Jenny Hsu, "HUD Releases Homelessness Report," *Journal of Housing & Community Development* 71, no. 6 (December 11, 2014): 18.
102. Christopher Jencks, *The Homeless* (Cambridge, MA: Harvard University Press, 1995).
103. William Avison, Jane D. McLeod, and Bernice A. Pescosolido, *Mental Health, Social Mirror* (New York: Springer Science & Business Media, 2007): 393.
104. David G. Phillips and Richard M. Alperin, *The Impact of Managed Care on the Practice of Psychotherapy: Innovations, Implementation and Controversy* (New York: Routledge, 2013).
105. I. D. Cummins, "Deinstitutionalisation; Mental Health Services in the Age of Neo-Liberalism," *Social Policy and Social Work in Transition* 1, no. 2 (November 2010): 55–74.
106. Stephen Pattison, *Pastoral Care and Liberation* (Cambridge; New York: Cambridge University Press, 1994): 102.
107. Ibid., 103.
108. Vilma Santiago-Irizarry, *Medicalizing Ethnicity: The Construction of Latino Identity in a Psychiatric Setting* (Ithaca, NY: Cornell University Press, 2001): 42.
109. This question comes from conversation with Bruce Rogers-Vaughn.
110. George Monbiot, "Sick of This Market-Driven World? You Should Be," *The Guardian*, August 5, 2014.

3 In Their Own Words: Mental Health Consumers, Survivors, and Ex-Patients

1. John Read, Richard P. Bentall, and Roar Fosse, "Time to Abandon the Bio-Bio-Bio Model of Psychosis: Exploring the Epigenetic and Psychological Mechanisms by Which Adverse Life Events Lead to Psychotic Symptoms," *Epidemiologia E Psichiatria Sociale* 18, no. 4 (December 2009): 299–310.
2. Linda Joy Morrison, *Talking Back to Psychiatry: The Psychiatric Consumer/Survivor/Ex-Patient Movement* (New York: Routledge, 2005).
3. Judi Chamberlin, *On Our Own: Patient-Controlled Alternatives to the Mental Health System* (New York: Hawthorn Books, 1978).
4. Ibid., 81.
5. Ibid., 38.
6. Ibid., 173.
7. Chava Finlker, "'We Do Not Want to Be Split Up from Our Family': Group Home Tenants amidst Land Use Conflict," in *Psychiatry Disrupted: Theorizing Resistance and Crafting the (R)evolution* (Montreal; Ithaca, NY: McGill-Queen's University Press, 2014): 100.
8. Jim Read, Jill Reynolds, and Open University, *Speaking Our Minds: An Anthology of Personal Experiences of Mental Distress and Its Consequences* (United Kingdom: The Open University, 1996).
9. Chamberlin, *On Our Own*, 15.
10. Ibid., 33.
11. Els van Dongen, *Worlds of Psychotic People : Wanderers, "Bricoleurs" and Strategists* (London: Routledge, 2004).
12. Ibid., 7.
13. Ibid., 8.
14. Ibid., 10.
15. Ibid., 150.
16. Donald Capps, *Fragile Connections: Memoirs of Mental Illness for Pastoral Care Professionals* (St Louis, MO: Chalice Press, 2005).
17. Linda Joy Morrison, *Talking Back to Psychiatry: The Psychiatric Consumer/survivor/ex-Patient Movement* (New York: Routledge, 2005): 58.
18. Phyllis Chesler, *Women and Madness* (San Diego: Harcourt Brace Jovanovich, 1989).
19. Morrison, *Talking Back to Psychiatry*, 67.
20. Ibid.
21. Ibid., 11.
22. Ibid., 79.
23. Ibid.
24. Ibid., 79.
25. Ted Curtis, Robert Dellar, and Leslie Esther, *Mad Pride*, Brentwood/Essex, UK: Chipmunkapublishing, 2011.

26. Morrison, *Talking Back to Psychiatry*, 17.
27. Ibid., 15.
28. Ibid., 11.
29. Ewen Speed, "Discourses of Acceptance and Resistance: Speaking Out about Psychiatry," in *De-Medicalizing Misery: Psychiatry, Psychology, and the Human Condition* (NY: Palgrave Macmillan, 2011): 129.
30. Morrison, *Talking Back to Psychiatry*, 93.
31. Rebecca Stringer, *Knowing Victims: Feminism, Agency and Victim Politics in Neoliberal Times* (Hove, East Sussex: Routledge, 2014).
32. Philip Thomas and Patrick J. Bracken, *Postpsychiatry* (Oxford; New York: Oxford University Press, 2005); Jim Read, Jill Reynolds, and Open University, *Speaking Our Minds*.
33. Thomas and Bracken, *Postpsychiatry*.
34. Morrison, *Talking Back to Psychiatry*, 153.
35. Morrison, *Talking Back to Psychiatry*.
36. Dongen, *Worlds of Psychotic People: Wanderers, "Bricoleurs" and Strategists*.
37. Morrison, *Talking Back to Psychiatry*, 109.
38. Ibid., 111.
39. Ibid., 110.
40. Ibid.
41. MindFreedom is the heir to the Mental Patients Liberation Front founded by Chamberlin and others.
42. Thomas and Bracken, *Postpsychiatry*, 81.
43. Prince, *Absent Citizens*.
44. John Swinton, "Building a Church for Strangers," *Journal of Religion, Disability, and Health*, 4/4 42.
45. Jim Read, Jill Reynolds, and Open University, *Speaking Our Minds*, 211.
46. Ibid., 209.
47. Ibid.
48. david, "The Highlander Statement of Concern and Call to Action March 25, 2000."
49. Morrison, *Talking Back to Psychiatry*, 92.
50. David Oaks, "The Highlander Statement of Concern and Call to Action March 25, 2000," *MFIPortal*. Accessed December 28, 2014.
51. Morrison, *Talking Back to Psychiatry*, 93.
52. Ibid.
53. David Epston and Michael White, *Narrative Means to Therapeutic Ends* (New York: Norton, 1990).
54. George Paulson, *Closing the Asylums: Causes and Consequences of the Deinstitutionalization Movement* (Jefferson, NC: McFarland, 2012).
55. Willie V. Bryan, *In Search of Freedom: How Persons with Disabilities Have Been Disenfranchised from the Mainstream of American Society and How the Search for Freedom Continues* (Springfield, IL: Charles C Thomas Publisher, 2006): 10.

56. Morrison, *Talking Back to Psychiatry*, 80.
57. Jim Read, Jill Reynolds, and Open University, *Speaking Our Minds*.
58. Thomas and Bracken, *Postpsychiatry*, 62.
59. Morrison, *Talking Back to Psychiatry*, 82.
60. Ibid.
61. David Reville, *Introducing Mad People's History*, 2010. https://www.youtube.com/watch?v=AKBFYi6A6pA&feature=youtube_gdata_player.
62. Morrison, *Talking Back to Psychiatry*, 81.
63. Ibid., 86.
64. Mick McKeown, Mark Cresswell, and Helen Spandler, "Deeply Engaged Relationships: Alliances between Mental Health Workers and Psychiatric Survivors in the U.K.," in *Psychiatry Disrupted: Theorizing Resistance and Crafting the (R)evolution* (Montreal: McGill-Queen's University Press, 2014): 152.
65. John Hopton and Vicki Coppock, *Critical Perspectives on Mental Health* (London; New York: Routlege, 2000): 50.
66. Alain Topor, *Managing The Contradictions: Recovery from Severe Mental Illness* (Saarbrücken: LAP Lambert Academic Publishing, 2012): 78.
67. Ibid.
68. Ibid., 179, emphasis mine.
69. Richard Warner, *Recovery from Schizophrenia: Psychiatry and Political Economy* (London; Boston: Routledge & Kegan Paul, 1985).
70. Els van Dongen, *Worlds of Psychotic People: Wanderers, "Bricoleurs" and Strategists* (London; New York: Routledge, 2004).
71. Thomas and Bracken, *Postpsychiatry*, 65.
72. Dongen, *Worlds of Psychotic People*.
73. Topor, *Managing The Contradictions*, 110.
74. Michael McCubbin and David Cohen, "Extremely Unbalanced: Interest Divergence and Power Disparties between Clients and Psychiatry." *International Journal of Law and Psychiatry* 19, no. 1 (1996): 1–25.
75. Marius Romme and Sandra Escher, eds., *Accepting Voices* (London: MIND, 1993).
76. Jim Read, Jill Reynolds, and Open University, *Speaking Our Minds*; Romme and Escher, *Accepting Voices*.
77. Thomas and Bracken, *Postpsychiatry*.
78. Romme and Escher, *Accepting Voices*.
79. Thomas and Bracken, *Postpsychiatry*, 66.
80. Bruce M. Z. Cohen, *Mental Health User Narratives: New Perspectives on Illness and Recovery* (Basingstoke, England; New York: Palgrave Macmillan, 2008): 103.
81. Cohen, *Mental Health User Narratives*.
82. Romme and Escher, *Accepting Voices*, 67.
83. Juli McGruder, "Madness in Zanzibar: An Exploration of Lived Experience," in *Schizophrenia, Culture, and Subjectivity: The Edge of Experience* (Cambridge: Cambridge University Press, 2004): 255–281.

84. Romme and Escher, *Accepting Voices*.
85. Jim Read, Jill Reynolds, and Open University, *Speaking Our Minds*, 27.
86. Romme and Escher, *Accepting Voices*, 59.
87. Ibid., 80.
88. Ibid., 81.
89. Romme and Escher, *Accepting Voices*; Jim Read, Jill Reynolds, and Open University, *Speaking Our Minds*.
90. Jim Read, Jill Reynolds, and Open University, *Speaking Our Minds*.
91. Thomas and Bracken, *Postpsychiatry*, 89.
92. Ibid., 77.
93. Ibid., 73.
94. Ibid., 104.
95. Ibid., 275.
96. Ibid., 108, 107.
97. Thomas, *The Dialectics of Schizophrenia*.
98. Ibid.
99. The Mental Health Foundation, *Strategies for Living* (London: Mental Health Foundation, 2000): 88.
100. Morrison, *Talking Back to Psychiatry*.
101. Judi Chamberlin, *On Our Own*.
102. Torbjörn Tännsjö, *Coercive Care: The Ethics of Choice in Health and Medicine* (London; New York: Routledge, 1999): 9.
103. Ibid., 43.
104. Ibid., 92.
105. Ibid., 7.
106. Chesler, *Women and Madness*.
107. Morrison, *Talking Back to Psychiatry*, 100.
108. Jeff Evans, "Psychiatric Advanced Directives Face Obstacles: Infrastructure to Uphold Plans' Legitimacy Often Does Not Exist or Is Circumvented by Conflicting Laws," *Clinical Psychiatry News*, February 2005..
109. Ibid.
110. Ibid.
111. E. S. Rogers et al., "A Consumer-Constructed Scale to Measure Empowerment among Users of Mental Health Services," *Psychiatric Services (Washington, D.C.)* 48, no. 8 (August 1997): 1042–1047.
112. David Reville, *Introducing Mad People's History*.
113. McKeown, Cresswell, and Spandler, "Deeply Engaged Relationships," 148.
114. Ibid., 151.
115. Ibid., 155.
116. Ibid., 157.
117. Randy Slorach, "Marxism and Disability," *International Journal of Socialism*, no. 129 (January 4, 2011).
118. Pembroke and Survivors Speak Out, *Self-Harm*, 13–15.

119. Mark Cresswell, "Psychiatric 'Survivors' and Testimonies of Self-Harm," *Social Science & Medicine* 61, no. 8 (October 2005): 1670.
120. Ibid., 1672.
121. Ibid., 1674.
122. Ibid., emphasis in the original.
123. Shelly Rambo, *Spirit and Trauma: A Theology of Remaining* (Louisville, KY: Westminster John Knox Press, 2010).
124. Pembroke and Survivors Speak Out, *Self-Harm*.
125. "Inverse Paranoia."
126. The Mental Health Foundation, *Strategies for Living*.
127. Ibid.

4 Pastoral Counseling and Social-Class Shame

1. This chapter tracks Christina's internal processing rather than Robert's because of the importance of counselors becoming aware of their own responses to social class.
2. *Two American Families*. Frontline. Documentary film. Accessed February 4, 2015.
3. Rev Jill Mcnish and Richard L. Dayringer, *Transforming Shame: A Pastoral Response* (Binghamton, NY: Routledge, 2004).
4. Lauren Marie Appio, "Poor and Working-Class Clients' Social Class-Related Experiences in Therapy," 2013. http://academiccommons.columbia.edu/catalog/ac:165253.
5. Paul W. Pruyser, *The Minister as Diagnostician: Personal Problems in Pastoral Perspective* (Philadelphia: Westminster John Knox Press, 1976).
6. This is not an actual diagnosis, but is fabricated to make a point about the importance of the social world.
7. Lisa A. Goodman et al., "Applying Feminist Theory to Community Practice," in *Advancing Social Justice through Clinical Practice* (Mahwah, NJ: Erlbaum, 2007): 260.
8. Bonnie Miller-McLemore, "The Living Human Web," in *Images of Pastoral Care: Classic Readings* (St. Louis, MO: Chalice Press, 2005): 60–67.
9. Joerg Rieger, *No Rising Tide: Theology, Economics, and the Future* (Minneapolis, MN: Fortress Press, 2009): 57.
10. Malinda Evans Hicks, "Reducing Disparities in the Use of Treatments for Depression and Other Mood Disorders." University of Texas, Dallas, 2013, Unpublished dissertation.
11. L. Townsend, *An Introduction to Pastoral Counseling* (Nashville, TN: Abingdon Press, 2009).
12. Pamela D. Couture, "The Social Gospel and Pastoral Care Today," in *The Social Gospel Today* (Louisville, KY: Westminster John Knox Press, 2001): 160–169.

13. Donald Capps, *Living Stories: Pastoral Counseling in Congregational Context* (Minneapolis, MN: Fortress Press, 1998): 11.
14. Carroll A. Watkins Ali, *Survival & Liberation: Pastoral Theology in African American Context* (St. Louis, MO: Chalice Press, 1999): 33.
15. Ibid.
16. bell hooks, *Where We Stand: Class Matters* (New York: Routledge, 2000).
17. Kirk A. Bingaman, *Treating the New Anxiety: A Cognitive-Theological Approach* (Lanham, MD: Jason Aronson, Inc., 2007): 134.
18. http://www.aapc.org/about-us/anti-racist-multicultural-competences/
19. Appio, "Poor and Working-Class Clients' Social Class-Related Experiences in Therapy."
20. Ibid., 203.
21. Nicholas Ladany and Maryann Krikorian, "Psychotherapy Process and Social Class," in *Oxford Handbook of Social Class in Counseling* (Oxford; New York: Oxford University Press, 2013): 123.
22. "Two American Families." Frontline. Documentary film. Accessed February 4, 2015.
23. Thomas M. Shapiro, *The Hidden Cost of Being African American: How Wealth Perpetuates Inequality* (New York: Oxford University Press, 2004).
24. Erik Olin Wright, *Approaches to Class Analysis* (Cambridge, UK; New York: Cambridge University Press, 2005): 22.
25. Ibid.
26. Ibid.
27. Barbara Ehrenreich, *Nickel and Dimed: On (Not) Getting by in America* (New York: Henry Holt & Co, 2008).
28. Wright, *Approaches to Class Analysis*, 20.
29. Rieger, *Religion, Theology, and Class: Fresh Engagements After Long Silence* (New York: Palgrave Macmillan, 2013).
30. Wright, *Approaches to Class Analysis*, 21.
31. Ladany and Krikorian, "Psychotherapy Process and Social Class," 123.
32. Ehrenreich, *Nickel and Dimed*.
33. Shapiro, *The Hidden Cost of Being African American*.
34. Rieger, *No Rising Tide*, 43.
35. Ibid., 57.
36. Ehrenreich, *Nickel and Dimed*.
37. Robert Walker, *The Shame of Poverty* (Oxford: Oxford University Press, 2014): 37.
38. Ibid., 82, 65.
39. Philip Browning Helsel, "Social Phobia and the Experience of Shame: Childhood Origins and Pastoral Implications," *Pastoral Psychology* 53, no. 6 (July 1, 2005): 535–540.
40. Gershen Kaufman, *Shame: The Power of Caring* (Rochester, VT: Schenkman Books, 1980).
41. Walker, *The Shame of Poverty*.

42. Rogers-Vaughn, "Blessed Are Those Who Mourn: Depression As Political Resistance," *Pastoral Psychology*, (2013): 511.
43. Kate Pickett and Richard Wilkinson, *The Spirit Level: Why Greater Equality Makes Societies Stronger*, reprint ed. (New York: Bloomsbury Press, 2011).
44. Rogers-Vaughn, "Blessed Are Those Who Mourn, 511.
45. Helsel, "Social Phobia and the Experience of Shame."
46. Thandeka, *Learning to Be White: Money, Race and God in America* (New York: Bloomsbury Academic, 2001): 3.
47. Walker, *The Shame of Poverty*.
48. Ibid., 128.
49. Ming Yan "Literature as a Window to Conceptions of Poverty and Shame in China" in *Poverty and Shame: Global Experiences* (Oxford: Oxford University Press, 2015).
50. Ehrenreich, *Nickel and Dimed*.
51. Walker, *The Shame of Poverty*, 128.
52. Elizabeth King Keenan, "Using Foucault's 'Disciplinary Power' and 'Resistance' in Cross-Cultural Psychotherapy," *Clinical Social Work Journal* 29, no. 3 (2001): 211; Patricia A. Joyce, "The Case Conference as Social Ritual Constructing a Mother of a Sexually Abused Child," *Qualitative Social Work* 4, no. 2 (June 1, 2005): 157–173.
53. Aaron T. Beck, *Anxiety Disorders and Phobias: A Cognitive Perspective*, 15th anniversary ed. (Cambridge, MA: Basic Books, 2005).
54. David Smail, *Power, Interest and Psychology* (Ross-on-Wye: PCCS Books, 2013); Ian Parker, *Revolution in Psychology: Alienation to Emancipation* (London: Pluto Press, 2007).
55. From a personal conversation with Ben Broderick, CBHI counselor.
56. Ali, *Survival & Liberation*.
57. Ramón Rojano, "The Practice of Community Family Therapy," in *Advancing Social Justice through Clinical Practice* (Mahwah, NJ: Erlbaum, 2007): 249, 252.
58. Ibid.
59. Ibid., 259.
60. Goodman et al., "Applying Feminist Theory to Community Practice."
61. Ibid.
62. Ibid., 275.
63. Helsel, "Definitional Ceremonies as Counter-Rituals to Case Conferences in Pastoral Care." *Practical Matters*, 7, April 2014.
64. Steven Friedman, *The Reflecting Team in Action: Collaborative Practice in Family Therapy* (New York: Guilford Press, 1995).
65. Eva Kjellberg et al., "Using the Reflecting Process with Families Stuck in Violence and Child Abuse," in *The Reflecting Team in Action* (New York: Guilford Press, 1998): 43.
66. Ibid., 43–44.
67. Ibid., 49.

68. Ibid., 51, 52.
69. Ibid., 54.
70. Ibid., 41.
71. Ibid., 44.
72. Rieger, *No Rising Tide*.
73. Couture, "The Social Gospel and Pastoral Care Today," 165.
74. Donal Dorr, *Option for the Poor and for the Earth: Catholic Social Teaching* (Maryknoll, NY: Orbis Books, 2012).
75. Ibid., 20th anniversary ed.: 4.
76. John A. Ryan, *Economic Justice: Selections from Distributive Justice and a Living Wage*, Library of Theological Ethics (Louisville, KY: Westminster John Knox Press, 1996).
77. Dorr, *Option for the Poor and for the Earth*.
78. Rieger, *No Rising Tide*, 70.
79. John Randall Sachs, *The Christian Vision of Humanity: Basic Christian Anthropology*. Zacchaeus Studies. Theology (Collegeville, MN: Liturgical Press, 1991): 8.
80. Gary J. Dorrien, *Reconstructing the Common Good: Theology and the Social Order* (Maryknoll, NY: Orbis Books, 1990).
81. Donald Capps, *Life Cycle Theory and Pastoral Care* (Eugene, OR: Wipf and Stock Publishers, 2002): 92.
82. Lawrence Holben, *All the Way to Heaven: The Selected Letters of Dorothy Day* (Milwaukee, WI: Marquette University Press, 2010).
83. Gustavo Gutierrez, "Liberation Theology and Activism," October 5, 2014.

5 The Counter-Conducts of Pastoral Power

1. Michel Foucault, *Security, Territory, Population: Lectures at the Collège de France 1977–1978* (New York: Picador, 2009); Matthew Chrulew, "Pastoral Counter-Conducts: Religious Resistance in Foucault's Genealogy of Christianity," *Critical Research on Religion* 2, no. 1 (April 1, 2014): 55–65; A. I. Davidson, "In Praise of Counter-Conduct," *History of the Human Sciences* 24, no. 4 (2011).
2. Jonathan Tran, *Foucault and Theology* (London; New York: T & T Clark, 2011): 1.
3. Janet Afary and Kevin B. Anderson, *Foucault and the Iranian Revolution: Gender and the Seductions of Islamism*, annotated ed. (Chicago: University of Chicago Press, 2005): 255.
4. Phiip S. Wang, Patricia A. Berglund, and Ronald C. Kessler, "Patterns and Correlates of Contacting Clergy for Mental Disorders in the United States," *Health Services Research* 38, no. 2 (April 2003): 647–673; Michael Moran et al., "A Study of Pastoral Care, Referral, and Consultation Practices Among Clergy in Four Settings in the New York City Area," *Pastoral Psychology* 53, no. 3 (January 1, 2005): 255–266.

5. Jan Hoffman, "More Pastors Embrace Talk of Mental Ills," *The New York Times*, November 28, 2014.
6. "24 Hours of Hope." Accessed March 7, 2015.
7. Plenary 1. *The Role of the Church in Mental Health—Rick Warren, Bishop Kevin Vann*, 2014. https://www.youtube.com/watch?v=zoxZjWuK2zA&feature=youtube_gdata_player.
8. Ibid.
9. Ibid.
10. Wang, Berglund, and Kessler, "Patterns and Correlates of Contacting Clergy for Mental Disorders in the United States."
11. Linda M. Chatters et al., "Use of Ministers for a Serious Personal Problem among African Americans: Findings from the National Survey of American Life." *The American Journal of Orthopsychiatry* 81, no. 1 (January 2011): 118–127.
12. Thomas Mackenzie and Christie Cozad Neuger, "Anxiety Disorders," in *Ministry with Persons with Mental Illness and Their Families* (Minneapolis, MN: Fortress Press, 2012): 33–57.
13. Bruce Curtis, "Foucault on Governmentality and Population: The Impossible Discovery," *The Canadian Journal of Sociology / Cahiers Canadiens de Sociologie* 27, no. 4 (October 1, 2002): 505–533; Jonathan Tran, *Foucault and Theology* (London; New York: T & T Clark, 2011). Curtis critiqued Foucault's elaboration of these concepts, offering additional clarity to describe them.
14. Foucault, *Security, Territory, Population*, 124.
15. Ibid., 128.
16. Ibid., 127.
17. William A. Clebsch, *Pastoral Care in Historical Perspective* (New York: J. Aronson, 1975): 4.
18. Seward Hiltner, *Preface to Pastoral Theology. The Ayer Lectures, 1954* (New York: Abingdon Press, 1958): 16.
19. Foucault, *Security, Territory, Population*, 127.
20. Ibid., 192.
21. Donald Capps, *Giving Counsel: A Minister's Guidebook* (St. Louis, MO: Chalice Press, 2001).
22. Ann Cvetkovich, *Depression: A Public Feeling* (Durham, NC; London: Duke University Press, 2012): 5.
23. David Smail, *Power, Interest and Psychology* (Ross-on-Wye: PCCS Books, 2013).
24. Foucault, *Security, Territory, Population*, 192.
25. William R. Crockett, *Eucharist, Symbol of Transformation* (New York: Pueblo, 1989).
26. Emmanuel Yartekwei Lartey, *In Living Colour: An Intercultural Approach to Pastoral Care and Counselling* (London; Herndon, VA: Cassell, 1997).
27. Joseph W. Ciarrocchi, *A Minister's Handbook of Mental Disorders* (Mahwah, NJ: Paulist Press, 1993): 67.

28. Cooper-White, *The Cry of Tamar: Violence against Women and the Church's Response* (Minneapolis, MN: Fortress Press, 2012).
29. Chrulew, "Pastoral Counter-Conducts"; Davidson, "In Praise of Counter-Conduct."
30. Foucault, *Security, Territory, Population*, 212.
31. Ibid., 213.
32. Thomas and Bracken, *Postpsychiatry*, 66.
33. John Swinton, "Dementia," presented at the Conference on Medicine and Religion (Chicago, IL, USA, May 28, 2013).
34. Swinton, *Resurrecting the Person: Friendship and the Care of People with Mental Health Problems* (Nashville, TN: Abingdon, 2000): 159.
35. Foucault, *Security, Territory, Population*, 210.
36. Ibid., 204. During the Reformation period infant baptism also implied civil identity since it was the time during which the name was given. Civil identity lead to forced military conscription, which this pacifist group rejected.
37. Ibid., 211.
38. Tran, *Foucault and Theology*, 6.
39. Bruce T. Morrill, *Anamnesis as Dangerous Memory: Political and Liturgical Theology in Dialogue* (Collegeville, MN: Liturgical Press, 2000).
40. Philip Goodchild, *Theology of Money* (Durham, NC: Duke University Press, 2009).
41. Joerg Rieger, *No Rising Tide: Theology, Economics, and the Future* (Minneapolis, MN: Fortress Press, 2009).
42. Lucy Atkinson Rose, *Sharing the Word:Preaching in the Roundtable Church* (Louisville, KY: Westminster John Knox Press, 1997); Letty M. Russell, *Church in the Round: Feminist Interpretation of the Church* (Louisville, KY: Westminster/JKnox Press, 1993).
43. Walter Brueggemann, *Struggling with Scripture* (Louisville, KY: Westminster John Knox Press, 2002).
44. Avaren Ipsen, *Sex Working and the Bible*. Bible World (London; Oakville, CT: Equinox Pub, 2009).
45. Brueggemann, *Struggling with Scripture*.
46. A. K. M. Adam, "Rhetoric, Postmodernism, and Theological Education: What Has Vincennes to Do with Athens or Jerusalem," in *To Teach, Delight, and to Move: Theological Education in a Post-Christian World* (Eugene, OR: Cascade Book, 2004): 71.
47. Foucault, *Security, Territory, Population*, 214.
48. Barbara Ehrenreich, *Nickel and Dimed, On (Not) Getting by in America* (New York: Henry Holt & Co, 2008): 68.
49. Dietrich Bonhoeffer, *Life Together, By Dietrich Bonhoeffer* (New York: Harper, 1954): 97.
50. Wayne E. Oates, *The Presence of God in Pastoral Counseling* (Waco, TX: Word Books, 1986): 123.

51. Joerg Rieger, *No Rising Tide: Theology, Economics, and the Future* (Minneapolis, MN: Fortress Press, 2009).
52. Rebecca Kathleen Huskey, *Paul Ricoeur on Hope: Expecting the Good* (New York: Peter Lang, 2009).
53. Philip Browning Helsel, "Re-Membering the Body of Christ: Historical Origins and Psychological Implications of the Doctrine of the Communion of Saints," in *Heaven, Hell, and the Afterlife* (Santa Barbara, CA: ABC-CLIO, 2013): 140–157.

6 An Integrative Vision for Pastoral Power

1. Axel Honneth and Nancy Fraser, *Redistribution or Recognition? A Political-Philosophical Exchange* (London; New York: Verso, 2003).
2. Diana, "Dave Ramsey Responds to Flak About His New Multi-Million Dollar Home." *Conservative Post*. Accessed March 9, 2015.
3. Jennie Weiss Block, *Copious Hosting: A Theology of Access for People with Disabilities* (New York: Continuum, 2002).
4. This is not to critique such efforts, but rather the role that they seem to play in addressing symptoms rather than getting at the root issues.
5. Erik Olin Wright, *Approaches to Class Analysis* (Cambridge, UK; New York: Cambridge University Press, 2005).
6. Block, *Copious Hosting*.
7. Frederick Solt, Philip Habel, and J. Tobin Grant, "Economic Inequality, Relative Power, and Religiosity," *Social Science Quarterly* 92, no. 2 (June 1, 2011): 447–465.
8. Dale B. Martin, *The Corinthian Body* (New Haven: Yale University Press, 1999): xvii.
9. Ibid.
10. Martin, *The Corinthian Body*.
11. Ibid., 95.
12. Ibid.
13. Tim Scott, Neil Stanford, and David R. Thompson, "Killing Me Softly: Myth in Pharmaceutical Advertising." *BMJ: British Medical Journal* 329, no. 7480 (December 18, 2004): 1484–1487.
14. Matt Bloom, "Are the Poor Happier? Perspectives from Business Management," in *The Preferential Option for the Poor Beyond Theology* (Notre Dame, IN: University of Notre Dame Press, 2014): 69–82.
15. Monika A. Bauer et al., "Cuing Consumerism Situational Materialism Undermines Personal and Social Well-Being," *Psychological Science* 23, no. 5 (May 1, 2012): 517–523.
16. Nick Hanauer, "The Pitchforks Are Coming... for Us Plutocrats," *POLITICO Magazine*. Accessed August 29, 2014.

17. Suniya S. Luthar and Shawn J. Latendresse, "Children of the Affluent," *Current Directions in Psychological Science* 14, no. 1 (February 2005): 49–53.
18. Ching Kwan Lee, *Against the Law: Labor Protests in China's Rustbelt and Sunbelt* (Oakland, CA: University of California Press, 2007): 169.
19. Richard Warner, *Recovery from Schizophrenia: Psychiatry and Political Economy* (London; Boston: Routledge & Kegan Paul, 1985).
20. Ethan Watters, *Crazy Like Us: The Globalization of the American Psyche*, reprint ed. (New York: Free Press, 2011).
21. Donald Capps, *Understanding Psychosis: Issues, Treatments, and Challenges for Sufferers and Their Families* (Blue Ridge Summit, PA: Rowman & Littlefield Publishers, 2014); Stewart D. Govig, *In the Shadow of Our Steeples: Pastoral Presence for Families Coping with Mental Illness* (New York: Routledge, 2000); *Strong at Broken Places: Persons with Disabilities and the Church* (Louisville, KY: Westminster John Knox Press, 1989).
22. Julie Holland, *Moody Bitches: The Truth About the Drugs You're Taking, The Sleep You're Missing, The Sex You're Not Having, and What's Really Making You Crazy* (New York: Penguin Press, 2015).
23. William Avison, Jane D. McLeod, and Bernice A. Pescosolido, *Mental Health, Social Mirror* (New York: Springer Science & Business Media, 2007).
24. Susan Dunlap, "Discourse Theory and Pastoral Theology," in *Feminist and Womanist Pastoral Theology* (Nashville: Abingdon Press, 1999): 133–148.
25. Jung Mo Sung, "Greed, Desire and Theology: Greed, Desire and Theology," *The Ecumenical Review* 63, no. 3 (October 2011): 251–262.
26. B. Rogers-Vaughn, "Blessed Are Those Who Mourn: Depression as Political Resistance," *Pastoral Psychology* (2013): 1–20.
27. Ramon Rójano, "The Practice of Community Family Therapy," in *Advancing Social Justice through Clinical Practice* (Mahwah, NJ: Erlbaum, 2007): 245–263.
28. David Harvey, *A Brief History of Neoliberalism* (Oxford; New York: Oxford University Press, 2005); Philip Goodchild, *Theology of Money* (Durham, NC: Duke University Press, 2009).
29. Chava Finlker, "'We Do Not Want to Be Split up from Our Family': Group Home Tenants amidst Land Use Conflict," in *Psychiatry Disrupted: Theorizing Resistance and Crafting the (R)evolution* (Montreal; Ithaca, NY: McGill-Queen's University Press, 2014): 96–113.
30. Jeff Evans, "Psychiatric Advanced Directives Face Obstacles: Infrastructure to Uphold Plans' Legitimacy Often Does Not Exist or Is Circumvented by Conflicting Laws," *Clinical Psychiatry News*, February 2005. Academic OneFile.
31. Thomas R. Cole, *No Color Is My Kind: The Life of Eldrewey Stearns and the Integration of Houston, Texas* (Austin: University of Texas Press, 1997).

32. Jim Read, Jill Reynolds, and Open University, *Speaking Our Minds. An Anthology of Personal Experiences of Mental Distress and Its Consequences* (United Kingdom: The Open University, 1996).
33. Philip Thomas and Patrick J. Bracken, *Postpsychiatry* (Oxford; New York: Oxford University Press, 2005): 77.
34. Cole, *No Color Is My Kind*, 10.
35. Ibid., 159.
36. Ibid., 161.
37. David Berman, *The Strange Demise of Jim Crow*. Documentary film.
38. Michel Foucault, *Power/Knowledge: Selected Interviews and Other Writings, 1972–1977* (New York: Pantheon Books, 1980): 81–82.
39. Mark Cresswell, "Psychiatric 'Survivors' and Testimonies of Self-Harm," *Social Science & Medicine* 61, no. 8 (October 2005): 1670.
40. E. S. Rogers et al., "A Consumer-Constructed Scale to Measure Empowerment among Users of Mental Health Services," *Psychiatric Services (Washington, D.C.)* 48, no. 8 (August 1997): 1042–1047.
41. Kathryn Doyle, "Living Wage Tied to Better Mental Health in London." *Reuters*. October 9, 2013.
42. Ken Untener, *The Practical Prophet, Pastoral Writings* (Mahwah, NJ: Paulist Press, 200): 1.

Bibliography

"24 Hours of Hope." Accessed March 7, 2015. http://mentalhealthandthechurch.com/Watch/Webcast/24-hours-of-hope.
"2014 Year-End U.S. Foreclosure Market Report | Newsroom and Media Center." Accessed March 10, 2015. http://www.realtytrac.com/news/foreclosure-trends/1-1-million-u-s-properties-with-foreclosure-filings-in-2014-down-18-percent-from-2013-to-lowest-level-since-2006/.
Aaron T. Beck. *Anxiety Disorders and Phobias: A Cognitive Perspective*. 15th anniversary ed. Cambridge, MA: Basic Books, 2005.
Adam, A. K. M. "Rhetoric, Postmodernism, and Theological Education: What Has Vincennes to Do with Athens or Jerusalem." In *To Teach, Delight, and To Move: Theological Education in a Post-Christian World*, 61–84. Eugene, OR: Cascade Book, 2004.
Afary, Janet, and Kevin B. Anderson. *Foucault and the Iranian Revolution: Gender and the Seductions of Islamism*. Annotated ed. Chicago: University Of Chicago Press, 2005.
Ali, Carroll A. Watkins. *Survival & Liberation: Pastoral Theology in African American Context*. St. Louis, MO: Chalice Press, 1999.
Allan V. Horwitz. *The Loss of Sadness: How Psychiatry Transformed Normal Sorrow into Depressive Disorder*. Oxford; New York: Oxford University Press, 2007.
Allen, Chris. "The Poverty of Death: Social Class, Urban Deprivation, and the Criminological Consequences of Sequestration of Death." *Mortality* 12, no. 1 (2007): 79–93. doi:10.1080/13576270601088392.
Allen, Theodore W., and State University of New York at Stony Brook Center for Study of Working Class Life. *Class Struggle and the Origin of Racial Slavery: The Invention of the White Race*. Center for the Study of Working Class Life, Dept. of Economics, State University of New York, 2006.
American Psychiatric Association. *Diagnostic and Statistical Manual of Mental Disorders*. DSM Library. American Psychiatric Association, 2013. http://dsm.psychiatryonline.org.proxy.bc.edu/doi/book/10.1176/appi.books.9780890425596.
Angell, Marcia. "Excess in the Pharmaceutical Industry." *CMAJ : Canadian Medical Association Journal* 171, no. 12 (December 7, 2004): 1451–1453. doi:10.1503/cmaj.1041594.

Appio, Lauren Marie. "Poor and Working-Class Clients' Social Class-Related Experiences in Therapy," 2013, unpublished dissertation. http://academiccommons.columbia.edu/catalog/ac:165253.

Asen, Robert. *Visions of Poverty: Welfare Policy and Political Imagination*. East Lansing, MI: MSU Press, 2012.

Avison, William, Jane D. McLeod, and Bernice A. Pescosolido. *Mental Health, Social Mirror*. New York: Springer Science & Business Media, 2007.

Bakunin, Mikhail Aleksandrovich. *Marxism, Freedom and the State*. Whitefish, MT: Kessinger Publishing, 2004.

Bassman, Ron. "Overcoming the Impossible" *Psychology Today* http://www.psychologytoday.com/articles/200101/overcoming-the-impossible, January 1, 2001.

Bauer, Monika A., James E. B. Wilkie, Jung K. Kim, and Galen V. Bodenhausen. "Cuing Consumerism Situational Materialism Undermines Personal and Social Well-Being." *Psychological Science* 23, no. 5 (May 1, 2012): 517–523. doi:10.1177/0956797611429579.

Berman, David. *The Strange Demise of Jim Crow*. Documentary film.

Biko, Steve. *I Write What I Like: Selected Writings*. Edited by Aelred Stubbs C. R. Chicago: University of Chicago Press, 2002.

Bingaman, Kirk A. *Treating the New Anxiety: A Cognitive-Theological Approach*. Lanham, MD: Jason Aronson, 2007.

Blazer, Dan G. *The Age of Melancholy: "Major Depression" and Its Social Origin*. New York: Routledge, 2005.

Block, Jennie Weiss. *Copious Hosting: A Theology of Access for People with Disabilities*. New York: Continuum, 2002.

Bloom, Matt. "Are the Poor Happier? Perspectives from Business Management." In *The Preferential Option for the Poor Beyond Theology*, 69–82. Notre Dame, IN: University of Notre Dame Press, 2014.

Blustein, David L., Saliha Kozan, and Alice Connors-Kellgren. "Unemployment and Underemployment: A Narrative Analysis about Loss." *Journal of Vocational Behavior* 82, no. 3 (June 2013): 256–265. doi:10.1016/j.jvb.2013.02.005.

Bridges, Sarah, and Richard Disney. "Debt and Depression." *Journal of Health Economics* 29, no. 3 (May 2010): 388–403. doi:10.1016/j.jhealeco.2010.02.003.

Brown, B. J., and Sally Baker. *Responsible Citizens: Individuals, Health and Policy under Neoliberalism*. London: Anthem Press, 2013.

Brown, George W., and Patricia M. Moran. "Single Mothers, Poverty and Depression." *Psychological Medicine* 27, no. 1 (January 1997): 21–33.

Brown, Sarah, Karl Taylor, and Stephen Wheatley Price. "Debt and Distress: Evaluating the Psychological Cost of Credit." *Journal of Economic Psychology* 26, no. 5 (2005): 642–663. doi:10.1016/j.joep.2005.01.002.

Bruce P. Dohrenwend Foundations' Fund for Research in Psychiatry Professor and Professor of Public Health Columbia University. *Adversity, Stress, and Psychopathology*. New York: Oxford University Press, 1998.

Brueggemann, Walter. *Struggling with Scripture*. Louisville, KY: Westminster John Knox Press, 2002.

Bryan, Willie V. *In Search of Freedom: How Persons with Disabilities Have Been Disenfranchised from the Mainstream of American Society and How the Search for Freedom Continues.* Springfield, IL: Charles C Thomas Publishers, 2006.

Bullock, Heather E. "Justifying Inequality: A Social Psychological Analysis of Beliefs about Poverty and the Poor." In *The Colors of Poverty: Why Racial and Ethnic Disparities Persist.* New York: Sage Publications, 2008.

"Bureau of Labor Statistics Data." Accessed January 12, 2015. http://data.bls.gov/timeseries/LNU04000000?years_option=all_years&periods_option=specific_periods&periods=Annual+Data.

Capps, Donald. *Fragile Connections: Memoirs of Mental Illness for Pastoral Care Professionals.* St Louis, MO: Chalice Press, 2005.

———. *Giving Counsel: A Minister's Guidebook.* St. Louis, MO: Chalice Press, 2001.

———. *Life Cycle Theory and Pastoral Care.* Eugene, OR: Wipf and Stock Publishers, 2002.

———. *Living Stories: Pastoral Counseling in Congregational Context.* Minneapolis, MN: Fortress Press, 1998.

———. *Understanding Psychosis: Issues, Treatments, and Challenges for Sufferers and Their Families.* Blue Ridge Summit, PA: Rowman & Littlefield Publishers, 2014.

Carroll, Jackson W. *God's Potters: Pastoral Leadership and the Shaping of Congregations.* Grand Rapids, MI: Wm. B. Eerdmans Publishing Company, 2006.

"CDC: Mental Disorders Rising in Children." Accessed February 6, 2015. http://www.ajc.com/news/news/cdc-mental-disorders-rising-in-children/nXs9f/

Center for Community Economic Development. "Closing the Racial Wealth Gap," October 27–29, 2007. http://www.insightcced.org/uploads/publications/assets/Insight_Convening_Report_Final_Public_Version.pdf

Chamberlin, Judi. *On Our Own: Patient-Controlled Alternatives to the Mental Health System.* New York: Hawthorn Books, 1978.

Charlton, James I. *Nothing about Us without Us: Disability Oppression and Empowerment.* Berkeley: University of California Press, 1998.

Chatters, Linda M., Jacqueline S. Mattis, Amanda Toler Woodward, Robert Joseph Taylor, Harold W. Neighbors, and Nyasha A. Grayman. "Use of Ministers for a Serious Personal Problem among African Americans: Findings from the National Survey of American Life." *The American Journal of Orthopsychiatry* 81, no. 1 (January 2011): 118–127. doi:10.1111/j.1939-0025.2010.01079.x.

Chesler, Phyllis. *Women and Madness.* San Diego: Harcourt Brace Jovanovich, 1989.

Chrulew, Matthew. "Pastoral Counter-Conducts: Religious Resistance in Foucault's Genealogy of Christianity." *Critical Research on Religion* 2, no. 1 (April 1, 2014): 55–65. doi:10.1177/2050303214520776.

Ciarrocchi, Joseph W. *A Minister's Handbook of Mental Disorders.* Mahwah, NJ: Paulist Press, 1993.

Clebsch, William A. *Pastoral Care in Historical Perspective.* New York: J. Aronson, 1975.

Cohen, Bruce M. Z. *Mental Health User Narratives: New Perspectives on Illness and Recovery*. Basingstoke, England; New York: Palgrave Macmillan, 2008.
Cole, Thomas R. *No Color Is My Kind: The Life of Eldrewey Stearns and the Integration of Houston, Texas*. Austin: University of Texas Press, 1997.
Conrad, Peter. *The Medicalization of Society: On the Transformation of Human Conditions into Treatable Disorders*. Baltimore: Johns Hopkins University Press, 2007.
Conrad, Peter, and Caitlin Slodden. "The Medicalization of Mental Disorder." In *Handbook of the Sociology of Mental Health*, 2nd ed., 61–73. New York: Springer, 2013.
Cooper, Melinda E. *Life as Surplus: Biotechnology and Capitalism in the Neoliberal Era*. Seattle: University of Washington Press, 2008.
Cooper-White, Pamela. *The Cry of Tamar: Violence against Women and the Church's Response*. Minneapolis, MN: Fortress Press, 2012.
Couldry, Nick. *Why Voice Matters: Culture and Politics After Neoliberalism*. London: Sage, 2010.
Couture, Pamela D. "The Social Gospel and Pastoral Care Today." In *The Social Gospel Today*, 160–169. Louisville, KY: Westminster John Knox Press, 2001.
Cox, Harvey. "The Market as God." *The Atlantic*, March 1999. http://www.theatlantic.com/magazine/archive/1999/03/the-market-as-god/306397/.
Crenshaw, Kimberle. "Mapping the Margins: Intersectionality, Identity Politics, and Violence against Women of Color." *Stanford Law Review* 43, no. 6 (July 1, 1991): 1241–1299. doi:10.2307/1229039.
Cresswell, Mark. "Psychiatric 'Survivors' and Testimonies of Self-Harm." *Social Science & Medicine* 61, no. 8 (October 2005): 1668–1677. doi:10.1016/j.socscimed.2005.03.033.
Crockett, William R. *Eucharist, Symbol of Transformation*. New York: Pueblo, 1989.
Cummins, I. D. "Deinstitutionalisation; Mental Health Services in the Age of Neo-Liberalism." *Social Policy and Social Work in Transition* 1, no. 2 (November 2010): 55–74.
Curtis, Bruce. "Foucault on Governmentality and Population: doi:10.2307/3341588.
Curtis, Ted, Robert Dellar, and Leslie Esther. *Mad Pride*. Brentwood/Essex, UK: Chipmunka Publishing, 2011.
Cushman, Philip. *Constructing the Self, Constructing America: A Cultural History of Psychotherapy*. Cambridge, MA: Da Capo Press, 1996.
Cvetkovich, Ann. *Depression: A Public Feeling*. Durham, NC; London: Duke University Press, 2012.
Davidson, A. I. "In Praise of Counter-Conduct." *History of the Human Sciences* 24, no. 4 (2011). doi:10.1177/0952695111411625.
Diana. "Dave Ramsey Responds to Flak About His New Multi-Million Dollar Home." *Conservative Post*. Accessed March 9, 2015. http://conservativepost.com/dave-ramsey-responds-to-flak-about-his-new-multi-million-dollar-home/.

Díaz, R. M., G. Ayala, E. Bein, J. Henne, and B. V. Marin. "The Impact of Homophobia, Poverty, and Racism on the Mental Health of Gay and Bisexual Latino Men: Findings from 3 US Cities." *American Journal of Public Health* 91, no. 6 (2001): 927.
Dietrich Bonhoeffer. *Life Together: By Dietrich Bonhoeffer*. New York: Harper, 1954.
Doehring, Carrie. *The Practice of Pastoral Care: A Postmodern Approach*. Louisville, KY: Westminster John Knox Press, 2006.
Dongen, Els van. *Worlds of Psychotic People: Wanderers, "Bricoleurs" and Strategists*. London; New York: Routledge, 2004.
Dorr, Donal. *Option for the Poor and for the Earth: Catholic Social Teaching*. 20th anniversary ed. Maryknoll, NY: Orbis Books, 2012.
Dorrien, Gary J. *Reconstructing the Common Good: Theology and the Social Order*. Maryknoll, NY: Orbis Books, 1990.
Doyle, Kathryn. "Living Wage Tied to Better Mental Health in London." *Reuters*. October 9, 2013. http://www.reuters.com/article/2013/10/09/us-living-wage-idUSBRE99817E20131009.
Drentea, Patricia, and John R. Reynolds. "Neither a Borrower Nor a Lender Be." *Journal of Aging and Health* 24, no. 4 (2012): 673–695. doi:10.1177/0898264311431304.
Duménil, Gérard. *The Crisis of Neoliberalism*. Reprint ed. Cambridge, MA: Harvard University Press, 2013.
Dunlap, Susan. "Discourse Theory and Pastoral Theology." In *Feminist and Womanist Pastoral Theology*, 133–148. Nashville, TN: Abingdon Press, 1999.
Eaton, William W., Carles Muntaner, Gregory Bovasso, and Corey Smith. "Socioeconomic Status and Depressive Syndrome: The Role of Inter- and Intra-Generational Mobility, Government Assistance, and Work Environment." *Journal of Health and Social Behavior* 42, no. 3 (September 1, 2001): 277–294. doi:10.2307/3090215.
"Economic Scarring: The Long-Term Impacts of the Recession." *Economic Policy Institute*. Accessed March 10, 2015. https://secure.epi.org/publication/bp243/.
Ehrenreich, Barbara. *Nickel and Dimed: On (Not) Getting by in America*. New York: Henry Holt & Co, 2008.
Epston, David, and Michael White. *Narrative Means to Therapeutic Ends*. New York: Norton, 1990.
Eugen Bleuler. *Dementia Praecox; Or, The Group of Schizophrenias*. Monograph Series on Schizophrenia; No. 1. New York, International Universities Press, 1950.
Evans, Jeff. "Psychiatric Advanced Directives Face Obstacles: Infrastructure to Uphold Plans' Legitimacy Often Does Not Exist or Is Circumvented by Conflicting Laws." *Clinical Psychiatry News*, February 2005. Academic OneFile.
Fanon, Frantz. *Black Skin, White Masks*. New York: Grove Press; Berkeley, CA, 2008.

Finlker, Chava. "'We Do Not Want to Be Split Up from Our Family': Group Home Tenants amidst Land Use Conflict." In *Psychiatry Disrupted: Theorizing Resistance and Crafting the (R)evolution*, 96–113. Montreal; Ithaca, NY: McGill-Queen's University Press, 2014.

Foucault, Michel. *The History of Sexuality*. New York: Vintage Books, 1990.

——. *Power/Knowledge: Selected Interviews and Other Writings, 1972–1977*. New York: Pantheon Books, 1980.

—— *Security, Territory, Population: Lectures at the Collège de France 1977–1978*. York: Picador, 2009.

Foundation, The Mental Health. *Strategies for Living*. London: Mental Health Foundation, 2000.

Friedman, Steven. *The Reflecting Team in Action: Collaborative Practice in Family Therapy*. New York: Guilford Press, 1995.

Fromm, Erich. *The Sane Society*. New York: Fawcett Premier, 1955.

Gabriel, Yiannis, David E. Gray, and Harshita Goregaokar. "Temporary Derailment or the End of the Line? Managers Coping with Unemployment at 50." *Organization Studies* 31, no. 12 (December 1, 2010): 1687–1712. doi:10.1177/0170840610387237.

Gans, Herbert. *The War against the Poor: The Underclass and Antipoverty Policy*. New York: Basic Books, 1996.

Gathergood, John. "Debt and Depression: Causal Links and Social Norm Effects." *The Economic Journal* 122, no. 563 (2012): 1094–1114. doi:10.1111/j.1468–0297.2012.02519.x.

Geddes, Jr, N. Freemantle, J. Mason, M. P. Eccles, and J. Boynton. "Selective Serotonin Reuptake Inhibitors (SSRIs) versus Other Antidepressants for Depression." In *The Cochrane Database of Systematic Reviews*. Hoboken, NJ: John Wiley & Sons, 1996. http://onlinelibrary.wiley.com/doi/10.1002/14651858.CD001851/abstract.

Goodchild, Philip. *Theology of Money*. Durham, NC: Duke University Press, 2009.

Goodman, Lisa A., Angela Litwin, Amanda Bohlig, Sarah R. Weintraub, Autumn Green, Joy Walker, Lucie White, and Nancy Ryan. "Applying Feminist Theory to Community Practice." In *Advancing Social Justice through Clinical Practice*, 265–290. Mahwah, NJ: Erlbaum, 2007.

Govig, Stewart D. *In the Shadow of Our Steeples: Pastoral Presence for Families Coping with Mental Illness*. New York: Routledge, 2000.

——. *Strong at Broken Places: Persons with Disabilities and the Church*. Louisville, KY: Westminster John Knox Press, 1989.

Greenberg, Gary. *The Book of Woe: The DSM and the Unmaking of Psychiatry*. New York: Blue Rider Press, a member of Penguin Group USA, 2013.

——. *Manufacturing Depression: The Secret History of a Modern Disease*. New York: Simon & Schuster, 2010.

Gula, Richard. *Just Ministry: Professional Ethics for Pastoral Ministers*. Mahwah: Paulist Press, 2010.

Gutierrez, Gustavo. "Liberation Theology and Activism." October 5, 2014.

Hanauer, Nick. "The Pitchforks Are Coming... for Us Plutocrats." *POLITICO Magazine*. Accessed August 29, 2014. http://www.politico.com/magazine/story/2014/06/the-pitchforks-are-coming-for-us-plutocrats-108014.html.
Harvey, David. *A Brief History of Neoliberalism*. Oxford; New York: Oxford University Press, 2005.
Hatcher, S. "Debt and Deliberate Self-Poisoning." *The British Journal of Psychiatry* 164, no. 1 (January 1, 1994): 111–114. doi:10.1192/bjp.164.1.111.
Healy, David. *The Antidepressant Era*. Reprint ed. Cambridge, MA: Harvard University Press, 1999.
Helsel, Philip Browning. "Definitional Ceremonies as Counter-Rituals to Case Conferences in Pastoral Care." *Practical Matters*, 7, April 2014.
―――. "Re-Membering the Body of Christ: Historical Origins and Psychological Implications of the Doctrine of the Communion of Saints." In *Heaven, Hell, and the Afterlife*, 140–157. Santa Barbara, CA: ABC-CLIO, 2013.
―――. "Social Phobia and the Experience of Shame: Childhood Origins and Pastoral Implications." *Pastoral Psychology* 53, no. 6 (July 1, 2005): 535–540. doi:10.1007/s11089-005-4819-3.
Henwood, Doug. "American Dream: It's Not Working." *Christianity and Crisis* 52, no. 9 (June 8, 1992): 195–197.
Hicks, Malinda Evans. "Reducing Disparities in the Use of Treatments for Depression and Other Mood Disorders." University of Texas, Dallas, 2013, unpublished dissertation.
Hiltner, Seward. *Preface to Pastoral Theology*. The Ayer Lectures, 1954. New York: Abingdon Press, 1958.
Hoffman, Jan. "More Pastors Embrace Talk of Mental Ills." *The New York Times*, November 28, 2014. http://www.nytimes.com/2014/11/29/health/more-pastors-embrace-talk-of-mental-ills.html.
Holben, Lawrence. *All the Way to Heaven: The Selected Letters of Dorothy Day*. Milwaukee, WI: Marquette University Press, 2010.
Holland, Julie. *Moody Bitches: The Truth About the Drugs You're Taking, The Sleep You're Missing, The Sex You're Not Having, and What's Really Making You Crazy*. New York: Penguin Press, 2015.
Honneth, Axel, and Nancy Fraser. *Redistribution or Recognition?: A Political-Philosophical Exchange*. London; New York: Verso, 2003.
hooks, bell. *Where We Stand: Class Matters*. New York: Routledge, 2000.
Hopton, John, and Vicki Coppock. *Critical Perspectives on Mental Health*. London; New York: Routlege, 2000.
Houle, Jason N. "Mental Health in the Foreclosure Crisis." *Social Science & Medicine* 118 (October 2014): 1–8. doi:10.1016/j.socscimed.2014.07.054.
Hsu, Jenny. "HUD Releases Homelessness Report." *Journal of Housing & Community Development* 71, no. 6 (December 11, 2014): 18.
Hunt, Matthew O. "Race/Ethnicity and Beliefs About Wealth and Poverty." *Social Science Quarterly* 85, no. 3 (September 2004): 827–853. doi:10.1111/j.0038-4941.2004.00247.x.

Huskey, Rebecca Kathleen. *Paul Ricoeur on Hope: Expecting the Good.* New York: Peter Lang, 2009.

Ipsen, Avaren. *Sex Working and the Bible.* Bible World, London; Oakville, CT: Equinox Pub, 2009.

Jencks, Christopher. *The Homeless.* Cambridge, MA: Harvard University Press, 1995.

Jim. "Inverse Paranoia," n.d.

Jones, Gavin Roger. *American Hungers: The Problem of Poverty in U.S. Literature, 1840–1945.* Princeton, NJ: Princeton University Press, 2008.

Jones, Nev, and Robyn Brown. "The Absence of Psychiatric C/S/X Perspectives in Academic Discourse: Consequences and Implications." *Disability Studies Quarterly* 33, no. 1 (December 18, 2012). http://dsq-sds.org/article/view/3433.

Joyce, Patricia A. "The Case Conference as Social Ritual Constructing a Mother of a Sexually Abused Child." *Qualitative Social Work* 4, no. 2 (June 1, 2005): 157–173. doi:10.1177/1473325005052391.

Karen Weise, "Bundled Mortgages Pose Problems for Housing Program." *ProPublica.* Accessed January 13, 2015. http://www.propublica.org/article/making-home-affordable-loan-modifications-denied-806.

Kaufman, Gershen. *Shame: The Power of Caring.* Rochester, VT: Schenkman Books, 1980.

Keenan, Elizabeth King. "Using Foucault's 'Disciplinary Power' and 'Resistance' in Cross-Cultural Psychotherapy." *Clinical Social Work Journal* 29, no. 3 (2001): 211.

Kjellberg, Eva, Margaretha Edwardsson, Birgitta Johansson Niemela, and Tomas Oberg. "Using the Reflecting Process with Families Stuck in Violence and Child Abuse." In *The Reflecting Team in Action,* 38–61. New York: Guilford Press, 1998.

Kleinman, Arthur. *Rethinking Psychiatry: From Cultural Category to Personal Experience.* New York; London: Free Press; Collier Macmillan, 1991.

Ladany, Nicholas, and Maryann Krikorian. "Psychotherapy Process and Social Class." In *Oxford Handbook of Social Class in Counseling,* 118–130. Oxford; New York: Oxford University Press, 2013.

Lamb, H. Richard, and Linda E. Weinberger. "Persons with Severe Mental Illness in Jails and Prisons: A Review." *Psychiatric Services* 49, no. 4 (April 1, 1998): 483–492. doi:10.1176/ps.49.4.483.

Lartey, Emmanuel Yartekwei. *In Living Colour: An Intercultural Approach to Pastoral Care and Counselling.* London; Herndon, VA: Cassell, 1997.

Lee, Ching Kwan. *Against the Law: Labor Protests in China's Rustbelt and Sunbelt.* Oakland, CA: University of California Press, 2007.

Lerner, Steve. *Sacrifice Zones: The Front Lines of Toxic Chemical Exposure in the United States.* Cambridge, MA: MIT Press, 2010.

Letty M. Russell. *Church in the Round: Feminist Interpretation of the Church.* Louisville, KY: Westminster/JKnox Press, 1993.

Levison, Jennifer Rebecca. "Elizabeth Parsons Ware Packard: An Advocate for Cultural, Religious, and Legal Change." *Alabama Law Review* 54 (2003, 2002): 985.
Lewis, Oscar. "The Culture of Poverty." *Society* 35, no. 2 (1998): 7–9. doi:10.1007/BF02838122.
Lin, Ann Chih, and David R. Harris. *The Colors of Poverty: Why Racial and Ethnic Disparities Persist.* New York: Russell Sage Foundation, 2008.
Lorant, V., D. Delige, W. Eaton, A. Robert, P. Philippot, and M. Ansseau. "Socioeconomic Inequalities in Depression: A Meta-Analysis." *American Journal of Epidemiology* 157, no. 2 (2003): 98–112.
Loring, M., and B. Powell. "Gender, Race and DSM-Iii: A Study of the Objectivity of Psychiatric Diagnostic Behavior." *Journal of Health and Social Behavior* 29, no. 1 (1988): 1–22.
Luthar, Suniya S., and Shawn J. Latendresse. "Children of the Affluent." *Current Directions in Psychological Science* 14, no. 1 (February 2005): 49–53. doi:10.1111/j.0963-7214.2005.00333.x.
Lynch, John W., George A. Kaplan, and Sarah J. Shema. "Cumulative Impact of Sustained Economic Hardship on Physical, Cognitive, Psychological, and Social Functioning." *New England Journal of Medicine* 337, no. 26 (December 25, 1997): 1889–1895. doi:10.1056/NEJM199712253372606.
Mackenzie, Thomas, and Christie Cozad Neuger. "Anxiety Disorders." In *Ministry with Persons with Mental Illness and Their Families*, 33–57. Minneapolis, MN: Fortress Press, 2012.
Mander, Jerry. *The Capitalism Papers: Fatal Flaws of an Obsolete System.* Berkeley, CA: Counterpoint, 2013.
Martin, Dale B. *The Corinthian Body.* New Haven: Yale University Press, 1999.
McClure, Barbara. *Moving Beyond Individualism in Pastoral Care and Counseling: Reflections on Theory, Theology, and Practice.* Eugene, OR: Cascade Books, 2010.
McCubbin, Michael, and David Cohen. "Extremely Unbalanced: Interest Divergence and Power Disparties between Clients and Psychiatry." *International Journal of Law and Psychiatry* 19, no. 1 (1996): 1–25. doi:10.1016/0160-2527(95)00028-3.
McGruder, Juli. "Madness in Zanzibar: An Exploration of Lived Experience." In *Schizophrenia, Culture, and Subjectivity: The Edge of Experience*, 255–281. Cambridge: Cambridge University Press, 2004.
McKeown, Mick, Mark Cresswell, and Helen Spandler. "Deeply Engaged Relationships: Alliances between Mental Health Workers and Psychiatric Survivors in the U.K." In *Psychiatry Disrupted: Theorizing Resistance and Crafting the (R)evolution*, 144–162. Montreal: McGill-Queen's University Press, 2014.
McLaughlin, K. A., A. Nandi, K. M. Keyes, M. Uddin, A. E. Aiello, S. Galea, and K. C. Koenen. "Home Foreclosure and Risk of Psychiatric Morbidity during the Recent Financial Crisis." *Psychological Medicine* 42, no. 07 (July 2012): 1441–1448. doi:10.1017/S0033291711002613.

Mcnish, Rev Jill, and Richard L. Dayringer. *Transforming Shame: A Pastoral Response.* Binghamton, NY: Routledge, 2004.

Meltzer, H., P. Bebbington, T. Brugha, R. Jenkins, S. McManus, and M. S. Dennis. "Personal Debt and Suicidal Ideation." *Psychological Medicine* 41, no. 4 (April 2011): 771–778. doi:10.1017/S0033291710001261.

Metzl, Jonathan. *The Protest Psychosis: How Schizophrenia Became a Black Disease.* Boston: Beacon Press, 2009.

Micale, Mark S., and Roy Porter. *Discovering the History of Psychiatry.* New York: Oxford University Press, 1994.

Miller-McLemore, Bonnie. "The Living Human Web." In *Images of Pastoral Care: Classic Readings*, 60–67. St. Louis, MO: Chalice Press, 2005.

Moffatt, Ken. "Surveillance and Government of the Welfare Recipient." In *Reading Foucault for Social Work*, 219–245. New York: Columbia University Press, 1999.

Monbiot, George. "Sick of This Market-Driven World? You Should Be." *The Guardian*, August 5, 2014. http://www.theguardian.com/commentisfree/2014/aug/05/neoliberalism-mental-health-rich-poverty-economy.

Moran, Michael, Kevin J. Flannelly, Andrew J. Weaver, Jon A. Overvold, Winifred Hess, and Jo Clare Wilson. "A Study of Pastoral Care, Referral, and Consultation Practices among Clergy in Four Settings in the New York City Area." *Pastoral Psychology* 53, no. 3 (January 1, 2005): 255–266. doi:10.1007/s11089-004-0556-3.

Morrill, Bruce T. *Anamnesis as Dangerous Memory: Political and Liturgical Theology in Dialogue.* Collegeville, MN: Liturgical Press, 2000.

Morrison, Linda Joy. *Talking Back to Psychiatry: The Psychiatric Consumer/Survivor/Ex-Patient Movement.* New York: Routledge, 2005.

Muntaner, Carles, Carme Borrell, and Haejoo Chung. "Class Relations, Economic Inequality and Mental Health: Why Social Class Matters to the Sociology of Mental Health." In *Mental Health, Social Mirror*, edited by William R. Avison, Jane D. McLeod, and Bernice A. Pescosolido, 127–141. Springer US, 2007. http://link.springer.com.proxy.bc.edu/chapter/10.1007/978-0-387-36320-2_6.

Muntaner, Carles, Carme Borrell, Haejoo Chung, Carl Cohen, and Sami Timimi. "Class Exploitation and Psychiatric Disorders: From Status Syndrome to Capitalist Syndrome." In *Liberatory Psychiatry*, 131–146. Cambridge, UK; New York: Cambridge University Press, 2008.

Muntaner, Carles, Carme Borrell, Judit Solà, Marc Marí-dell'olmo, Haejoo Chung, Maica Rodríguez-sanz, Joan Benach, Kátia B. Rocha, and Edwin Ng. "Class Relations and All-Cause Mortality: A Test of Wright's Social Class Scheme Using the Barcelona 2000 Health Interview Survey." *International Journal of Health Services: Planning, Administration, Evaluation* 41, no. 3 (2011): 431–458.

Muntaner, Carles, William W. Eaton, Richard Miech, and Patricia O'Campo. "Socioeconomic Position and Major Mental Disorders." *Epidemiologic Reviews* 26, no. 1 (2004): 53–62. doi:10.1093/epirev/mxh001.

Muntaner, C., W. W. Eaton, C. Diala, R. C. Kessler, and P. D. Sorlie. "Social Class, Assets, Organizational Control and the Prevalence of Common Groups of Psychiatric Disorders." *Social Science & Medicine* 47, no. 12 (1998): 2043–2053. doi:10.1016/S0277-9536(98)00309-8.

Myrdal, Gunnar. *Challenge to Affluence*. New York: Random House, 1963.

Nemec, Patricia B., LeRoy Spaniol, and Arthur E. Dell Orto. "Psychiatric Rehabilitation Education." *Rehabilitation Education* 15, no. 2 (n.d.).

Oaks, David. "The Highlander Statement of Concern and Call to Action March 25, 2000." *MFIPortal*. Accessed December 28, 2014. http://www.mindfreedom.org/kb/history/highlander-2000.

Oates, Wayne E. *The Presence of God in Pastoral Counseling*. Waco, TX: Word Books, 1986.

O'Brien, Gordon E. *Psychology of Work and Unemployment*. Vol. xiii. Wiley Series in Psychology and Productivity at Work. Oxford, England: John Wiley & Sons, 1986.

O'Connor, Alice. *Poverty Knowledge: Social Science, Social Policy, and the Poor in Twentieth-Century U.S. History*. Reprint ed. Princeton, NJ: Princeton University Press, 2002.

Office, US Census Bureau Public Information. "Nearly 1 in 5 People Have a Disability in the U.S., Census Bureau Reports—Miscellaneous—Newsroom—U.S. Census Bureau." Accessed March 10, 2015. https://www.census.gov/newsroom/releases/archives/miscellaneous/cb12-134.html.

Pantazis, Christina, David Gordon, and Ruth Levitas. *Poverty and Social Exclusion in Britain: The Millennium Survey*. Bristol, UK: Policy Press, 2006.

Parker, Ian. *Revolution in Psychology: Alienation to Emancipation*. London: Pluto Press, 2007.

"Part 1, How Mad Are You? 2008–2009, Horizon—BBC Two." *BBC*. Accessed February 6, 2015. http://www.bbc.co.uk/programmes/b00fm5ql.

Patnaik, Prabhat. *Retreat to Unfreedom: Essays on the Emerging World Order*. New Delhi: Tulika, 2003.

Pattison, Stephen. *Pastoral Care and Liberation*. Cambridge; New York: Cambridge University Press, 1994.

Patton, John. *Pastoral Care in Context: An Introduction to Pastoral Care*. Louisville, KY: Westminster/John Knox Press, 1993.

Paul, Karsten I., and Klaus Moser. "Unemployment Impairs Mental Health: Meta-Analyses." *Journal of Vocational Behavior* 74, no. 3 (2009): 264–282. doi:10.1016/j.jvb.2009.01.001.

Paulson, George. *Closing the Asylums: Causes and Consequences of the Deinstitutionalization Movement*. Jefferson, NC: McFarland, 2012.

Pembroke, Louise Roxanne, and Survivors Speak Out. *Self-Harm: Perspectives from Personal Experience*. London: Survivors Speak Out, 1996.

Perrucci, Robert. *The New Class Society: Goodbye American Dream?* 3rd ed. Lanham: Rowman & Littlefield Publishers, 2007.

Phillips, David G., and Richard M. Alperin. *The Impact of Managed Care on the Practice of Psychotherapy: Innovations, Implementation and Controversy.* New York: Routledge, 2013.

Pickett, Kate, and Richard Wilkinson. *The Spirit Level: Why Greater Equality Makes Societies Stronger.* Reprint ed. New York: Bloomsbury Press, 2011.

Plenary 1: The Role of the Church in Mental Health—Rick Warren, Bishop Kevin Vann, 2014. https://www.youtube.com/watch?v=zoxZjWuK2zA&feature=youtube_gdata_player.

Presbyterian Church. "Presbyterian Church (U.S.A.)—News & Announcements—Moonlighting Pastors and Postponed Health Care," April 8, 2014. http://www.pcusa.org/news/2014/4/8/moonlighting-pastors-and-postponed-health-care/.

Price, Richard H., Jin Nam Choi, and Amiram D. Vinokur. "Links in the Chain of Adversity Following Job Loss: How Financial Strain and Loss of Personal Control Lead to Depression, Impaired Functioning, and Poor Health." *Journal of Occupational Health Psychology* 7, no. 4 (October 2002): 302–312. doi:http://dx.doi.org.proxy.bc.edu/10.1037/1076-8998.7.4.302.

Prince, Michael J. *Absent Citizens: Disability Politics and Policy in Canada.* Toronto: University of Toronto Press, 2009.

Pruyser, Paul W. *The Minister as Diagnostician: Personal Problems in Pastoral Perspective.* Philadelphia: Westminster John Knox Press, 1976.

Putnam, Robert. *Our Kids: The American Dream in Crisis.* New York: Simon and Schuster, 2015.

"QuickStats: Prevalence of Current Depression among Persons Aged ≥12 Years, by Age Group and Sex—United States, National Health and Nutrition Examination Survey, 2007–2010." Accessed February 6, 2015. http://www.cdc.gov/mmwr/preview/mmwrhtml/mm6051a7.htm.

Rambo, Shelly. *Spirit and Trauma: A Theology of Remaining.* Louisville, KY: Westminster John Knox Press, 2010.

Raphael, Steven, and Michael A. Stoll. *Why Are So Many Americans in Prison?* New York: Russell Sage Foundation, 2013.

Razinsky, Liran. *Freud, Psychoanalysis and Death.* Cambridge, UK: Cambridge University Press, 2013.

Read, Jim, Jill Reynolds, and Open University. *Speaking Our Minds: An Anthology of Personal Experiences of Mental Distress and Its Consequences.* United Kingdom: The Open University, 1996.

Read, John, Richard P. Bentall, and Roar Fosse. "Time to Abandon the Bio-Bio-Bio Model of Psychosis: Exploring the Epigenetic and Psychological Mechanisms by Which Adverse Life Events Lead to Psychotic Symptoms." *Epidemiologia E Psichiatria Sociale* 18, no. 4 (December 2009): 299–310.

Reininghaus, Ulrich A., Craig Morgan, Jayne Simpson, Paola Dazzan, Kevin Morgan, Gillian A. Doody, Dinesh Bhugra, et al. "Unemployment, Social Isolation, Achievement–Expectation Mismatch and Psychosis: Findings from the ÆSOP Study." *Social Psychiatry and Psychiatric Epidemiology* 43, no. 9 (September 1, 2008): 743–751. doi:10.1007/s00127-008-0359-4.

Report Shows Racial Wealth Gap Widening.(13:00–14:00 PM)(an Insight Center for Community Economic Development report)(Broadcast transcript)(Audio File), 2010.

Reville, David. *Introducing Mad People's History*, 2010. https://www.youtube.com/watch?v=AKBFYi6A6pA&feature=youtube_gdata_player.

Rieger, Joerg. *No Rising Tide: Theology, Economics, and the Future*. Minneapolis, MN: Fortress Press, 2009.

———. *Religion, Theology, and Class: Fresh Engagements After Long Silence*. New York: Palgrave Macmillan, 2013.

Robert Walker. *The Shame of Poverty*. Oxford: Oxford University Press, 2014.

Rogers, E. S., J. Chamberlin, M. L. Ellison, and T. Crean. "A Consumer-Constructed Scale to Measure Empowerment among Users of Mental Health Services." *Psychiatric Services (Washington, D.C.)* 48, no. 8 (August 1997): 1042–1047.

Rogers-Vaughn, B. "Blessed Are Those Who Mourn: Depression As Political Resistance." *Pastoral Psychology* (2013): 1–20.

Rójano, Ramon. "The Practice of Community Family Therapy." In *Advancing Social Justice through Clinical Practice*, 245–263. Mahwah, NJ: Erlbaum, 2007.

Romme, Marius, and Sandra Escher, eds. *Accepting Voices*. London: MIND, 1993.

Rose, Lucy Atkinson. *Sharing the Word: Preaching in the Roundtable Church*. Louisville, KY: Westminster John Knox Press, 1997.

Rose, Nikolas S. *Governing the Soul: The Shaping of the Private Self*. London; New York: Routledge, 1990.

Rosenhan, David L. "On Being Sane in Insane Places." *Science: New Series* 179, no. 4070 (1973): 250–258.

Ryan, Jake, and Charles Sackrey. *Strangers in Paradise: Academics from the Working Class*. 2nd ed. Lanham: University Press of America, 1995.

Ryan, John A. *Economic Justice: Selections from Distributive Justice and a Living Wage*. Library of Theological Ethics. Louisville, KY: Westminster John Knox Press, 1996.

Sachs, John Randall. *The Christian Vision of Humanity: Basic Christian Anthropology*. Zacchaeus Studies. Theology. Collegeville, MN: Liturgical Press, 1991.

Sadeh, Noa, and Rachel Karniol. "The Sense of Self-Continuity as a Resource in Adaptive Coping with Job Loss." *Journal of Vocational Behavior* 80, no. 1 (February 2012): 93–99. doi:10.1016/j.jvb.2011.04.009.

Santiago-Irizarry, Vilma. *Medicalizing Ethnicity: The Construction of Latino Identity in a Psychiatric Setting*. Ithaca, NY: Cornell University Press, 2001.

Scott, Tim, Neil Stanford, and David R. Thompson. "Killing Me Softly: Myth in Pharmaceutical Advertising." *BMJ: British Medical Journal* 329, no. 7480 (December 18, 2004): 1484–1487.

Selenko, Eva, and Bernad Batinic. "Beyond Debt. A Moderator Analysis of the Relationship between Perceived Financial Strain and Mental Health." *Social Science & Medicine* 73, no. 12 (December 2011): 1725–1732. doi:10.1016/j.socscimed.2011.09.022.

Sennett, Richard. *The Hidden Injuries of Class*. New York: Knopf, 1972.
Service, Katherine Burgess| Religion News. "Report: Church Giving Reaches Depression-Era Record Lows." *The Washington Post*, October 24, 2013. http://www.washingtonpost.com/national/on-faith/report-church-giving-reaches-depression-era-record-lows/2013/10/24/b2721a56-3ce9-11e3-b0e7-716179a2c2c7_story.html.
Shapiro, Thomas M. *The Hidden Cost of Being African American: How Wealth Perpetuates Inequality*. New York: Oxford University Press, 2004.
Shin, Hyon-Uk. *Vulnerability and Courage a Pastoral Theology of Poverty and the Alienated Self*. New York: Peter Lang, 2012.
Slorach, Randy. "Marxism and Disability." *International Journal of Socialism*, no. 129 (January 4, 2011). http://www.isj.org.uk/?id=702#129slorach_45.
Smail, David. *Power, Interest and Psychology*. Ross-on-Wye: PCCS Books, 2013.
Solt, Frederick, Philip Habel, and J. Tobin Grant. "Economic Inequality, Relative Power, and Religiosity." *Social Science Quarterly* 92, no. 2 (June 1, 2011): 447–465. doi:10.1111/j.1540–6237.2011.00777.x.
Speed, Ewen. "Discourses of Acceptance and Resistance: Speaking Out about Psychiatry." In *De-Medicalizing Misery: Psychiatry, Psychology, and the Human Condition*, 123–140. New York: Palgrave Macmillan, 2011.
Stack, Steven, and Ira Wasserman. "Economic Strain and Suicide Risk: A Qualitative Analysis." *Suicide and Life-Threatening Behavior* 37, no. 1 (2007): 103–112. doi:10.1521/suli.2007.37.1.103.
Steinberg, Michael K., Joseph J Hobbs (Joseph John), and Kent Mathewson. *Dangerous Harvest: Drug Plants and the Transformation of Indigenous Landscapes*. New York: Oxford University Press, 2004.
Stringer, Rebecca. *Knowing Victims: Feminism, Agency and Victim Politics in Neoliberal Times*. Hove, East Sussex: Routledge, 2014.
Sung, Jung Mo. "Greed, Desire and Theology: Greed, Desire and Theology." *The Ecumenical Review* 63, no. 3 (October 2011): 251–262. doi:10.1111/j.1758–6623. 2011.00119.x.
Swinton, John. "Dementia." Presented at the Conference on Medicine and Religion, Chicago, IL, USA, May 28, 2013.
———. *Resurrecting the Person: Friendship and the Care of Persons with Mental Health Problems*. Nashville, TN: Abingdon Press, 2000.
———. "Building a Church for Strangers," *Journal of Religion, Disability, and Health*, 4/4: 26–63.
Szasz, Thomas. *The Myth of Mental Illness: Foundations of a Theory of Personal Conduct*. Revised ed. New York, Harper & Row, 1974.
———. "Varieties of Psychiatric Criticism." *History of Psychiatry* 23, no. 3 (September 1, 2012): 349–355. doi:10.1177/0957154X12450236.
Thandeka. *Learning to Be White: Money, Race and God in America*. New York: Bloomsbury Academic, 2001.
"The Best—and Worst—Places to Lose Your Job." *BBC Capital*. Accessed March 10, 2015. http://www.bbc.com/capital/story/20141217-the-worst-countries-for-sacking.

"The Pseudo-Patient Study, Mind Changers—BBC Radio 4." *BBC.* Accessed February 6, 2015. http://www.bbc.co.uk/programmes/b00lny48.
Thomas, Philip. *The Dialectics of Schizophrenia.* London; New York: Free Association Books, 1997.
Thomas, Philip, and Patrick J. Bracken. *Postpsychiatry.* Oxford; New York: Oxford University Press, 2005.
Topor, Alain. *Managing The Contradictions: Recovery from Severe Mental Illness.* Saarbrücken: LAP Lambert Academic Publishing, 2012.
Torbjörn Tännsjö. *Coercive Care: The Ethics of Choice in Health and Medicine.* London; New York: Routledge, 1999.
Townsend, L. *An Introduction to Pastoral Counseling.* Nashville, TN: Abingdon Press, 2009.
Tran, Jonathan. *Foucault and Theology.* London; New York: T & T Clark, 2011.
Turunen, Elina, and Heikki Hiilamo. "Health Effects of Indebtedness: A Systematic Review." *BMC Public Health* 14, no. 1 (May 22, 2014): 489. doi:10.1186/1471-2458-14-489.
Two American Families. Frontline. Documentary film. Accessed February 4, 2015. http://www.pbs.org/wgbh/pages/frontline/two-american-families/.
Untener, Ken. *The Practical Prophet: Pastoral Writings.* Mahwah, NJ: Paulist Press, 2007.
U'Ren, Richard. *Social Perspective: The Missing Element in Mental Health Practice.* Toronto; Buffalo: University of Toronto Press, Scholarly Publishing Division, 2011.
"USDA Economic Research Service—Geography of Poverty." Accessed February 21, 2015. http://www.ers.usda.gov/topics/rural-economy-population/rural-poverty-well-being/geography-of-poverty.aspx.
Walker, Carl, *Depression and Globalization: The Politics of Mental Health in the 21st Century.* New York: Springer, 2008.
Wanberg, Connie R. "The Individual Experience of Unemployment." *Annual Review of Psychology* 63, no. 1 (2012): 369–396. doi:10.1146/annurev-psych-120710-100500.
Wang, Philip S., Patricia A. Berglund, and Ronald C. Kessler. "Patterns and Correlates of Contacting Clergy for Mental Disorders in the United States." *Health Services Research* 38, no. 2 (April 2003): 647–673. doi:10.1111/1475-6773.00138.
Warner, Richard. *Recovery from Schizophrenia: Psychiatry and Political Economy.* London; Boston: Routledge & Kegan Paul, 1985.
Watters, Ethan. *Crazy Like Us: The Globalization of the American Psyche.* Reprint ed. New York: Free Press, 2011.
Weich, S., and G. Lewis. "Material Standard of Living, Social Class, and the Prevalence of the Common Mental Disorders in Great Britain." *Journal of Epidemiology and Community Health* 52, no. 1 (January 1, 1998): 8–14. doi:10.1136/jech.52.1.8.
White, Michael. *Narratives of Therapists' Lives.* Adelaide, South Australia: Dulwich Centre Publications, 1997.

Wright, Erik Olin. *Approaches to Class Analysis*. Cambridge, UK; New York: Cambridge University Press, 2005.
———. *Class Counts: Comparative Studies in Class Analysis*. Cambridge; New York: Paris: Cambridge University Press, 1996.
———. *Envisioning Real Utopias*. London; New York: Verso, 2010.
Yan, Ming. "Literature as a Window to Conceptions of Poverty and Shame in China." In *Poverty and Shame: Global Experiences,* edited by Elain Chase and Grace Bantebya-Kyomuhendo, 60–72. Oxford: Oxford University Press, 2014.

Index

advertising, 4, 7, 67, 69–70, 80, 191, 193
Agamben, Giorgio, 116
American Psychiatric Association (APA), 57, 63
Angell, Marcia, 62
antidepressants, 4, 61–3
Appio, Lauren Marie, 128
asceticism, 171–2
Association of Pastoral Counselors (AAPC), 126, 128, 153

Bassman, Ronald, 90, 93–5
Bauman, Zygmunt, 35, 152
Beck, Aaron, 141
Beck Depression Inventory, 141
Beresford, Peter, 93
Bingaman, Kirk, 127
bipolar disorder, 63, 168, 200
Black Skin, White Masks (Fanon), 65
Blazer, Dan, 63, 65
Bonhoeffer, Dietrich, 178
Budd, Su, 87
Bullock, Heather E., 38–9, 41

capitalism
  critique of, 41
  c/s/x activism and, 198
  disability and, 114
  exploitation and, 36
  Fromm on, 67–8
  injustice and, 149
  mental suffering and, 105–7, 119, 145, 180
  ministry and, 148, 171, 186
  neoliberalism and, 41, 43–4, 68, 156, 174
  Pattison on, 76
  rights and, 132
  social class and, 5, 31, 34–7
  Wright on, 44
Capps, Donald, 126, 151
Carroll, Jackson, 48
Carter, Jimmy, 74
Chabasinki, Ted, 92
Chamberlin, Judi, 83–8, 90, 92, 95–6, 99, 102, 112
Charcot, Jean-Martin, 66
Chesler, Phyllis, 87
civil rights, 82, 86, 104
coercive psychiatry, 66, 89, 98, 108–12
Cognitive Behavioral Therapy (CBT), 141–3
Cole, Thomas, 199–200
collective unconscious, 66
community, 168–71
Community Family Therapy (CFT), 144
Community Mental Health Act (1963), 74
Conference on Human Rights and Psychiatric Oppression, 87, 98
Congress on Hispanic Mental Health (CHMH), 70

Conrad, Peter, 58
consumers
 activism, 119
 advertising and, 4, 193
 advocacy and, 82
 explained, 13
 language and, 89–90
 mental illness and, 106, 158
 ministry and, 119
 narratives, 81
 rights movement, 95–100
 self-definition and, 197
 shame and, 9
 see also c/s/x movement
contradictory class location, 32, 124, 140
contradictory class position, 32, 34, 49–50, 148, 162–3, 171
Cooper, Melinda E., 25
Couture, Pamela, 149
Crenshaw, Kimberlé, 36
Cresswell, Mark, 116–17, 179
criminalization, 13, 78
c/s/x movement
 capitalism and, 198
 coercive psychiatry and, 108, 110
 disability and, 83, 92–3, 96, 114–15
 epistemology and, 13, 82, 98
 hearing voices and, 103–7
 identity and, 94, 97, 108
 MNN and, 87–90
 overview, 13–14, 16–17, 80, 82–3
 partnership and, 115–19
 poverty and, 105–6
 psychiatry and, 85–6
 rights and, 92–3
 self-definition and, 81, 83, 89, 107
 self-determination and, 13, 17, 81–2, 85–7, 89, 107
 themes and controversies in, 86–7
 see also consumers; ex-patients; literature, c/s/x movement; survivors

Cushman, Philip, 9
Cvetcovich, Ann, 4, 8, 160, 204n14

debt, 24–5
deinstitutionalization, 16, 41, 73–7, 88, 110, 114, 193, 197
 see also institutionalization; transinstitutionalization
Dershowitz, Alan, 108
Diagnostic and Statistical Manual of Mental Disorders (DSM-III), 55, 58–9, 63–5, 69–70, 72, 75, 86, 102, 124
disability
 capitalism and, 114
 children and, 127
 c/s/x activism and, 83, 92–3, 96, 114–15
 deinstitutionalization and, 74
 exclusion and, 35–7
 identity and, 92, 168
 mental health and, 11–13, 93–4
 ministry and, 185–6
 neoliberalism and, 37
 rights and, 93–4
 social, 93, 109, 114
 social class and, 33
Doehring, Carrie, 216n92

economic conditions, mental illness and
 debt, 24–5
 foreclosure, 25–6
 overview, 21–3
 unemployment, 23–4
ECT
 see shock therapy
Ehrenreich, Barbara, 135, 175
epistemology
 c/s/x activism and, 13, 82, 98
 mental illness and, 13, 63
 ministry and, 78, 190
 NAMI and, 98
 psychiatry and, 78–9, 107

eschatology, 174–6
ex-patients
 explained, 13, 82
 hearing voices and, 103, 105–6
 language and, 89–90
 narratives, 100–2
 pastoral counseling and, 119
 self-definition and, 197
 self-help groups and, 84
 see also c/s/x movement

Fanon, Frantz, 65–6, 68, 104
Felman, Shoshanna, 116
Foner, Janet, 87
foreclosures, 25–6
Foucault, Michel, 5, 14, 16, 45–6, 55–7, 87, 140, 156–7, 159–66, 170–2, 175, 184, 200
Frank, Leonard Roy, 87
Fromm, Erich, 67–8

Gans, Herbert, 40–1
gay and lesbian rights, 87–8, 93
Gifford, Gloria, 93
Gladden, Washington, 149
Global Assessment of Functioning (GAF), 75
globalization, 2, 20, 30, 47, 68, 130, 192
Great Recession, 23–4, 26, 29, 50
Greenberg, Gary, 60
Gross Domestic Product (GDP), 19, 24
Gutiérrez, Gustavo, 152

Hanauer, Sean, 191
Hanson, Janet Adair, 161
Harrison, Chris, 93
Harvey, David, 3
health maintenance organizations (HMOs), 75
Healy, David, 62, 64
hearing voices, 102–8, 119, 185
Hertz, Thomas, 134
History of Sexuality, The (Foucault), 159

homophobia, 21
hooks, bell, 8–9, 89, 111
Housing and Urban Development, 74
Howie the Harp, 87
Hunt, Matthew O., 38

impairment, 24, 93, 114
institutionalization, 13, 41, 73
 see also deinstitutionalization; transinstitutionalization
International Classification or Diseases (ICD), 59
Ionia State Hospital for the Criminally Insane, 69–70
Ipsen, Avaren, 174

jails
 see prisons
John of Chrysostom, 160
Jung, Karl, 66

Kaufman, Gershen, 136
Kennedy, John F., 74
Kleinman, Arthur, 55, 101
Kraepelin, Emil, 59–60, 63, 65, 69
Kramer, Peter, 61, 68

Lartey, Emmanuel, 163
Laub, Dori, 116
Learning to be White (Thandeka), 137
Lehrbuch fur Psychiatry (Kraepelin), 59, 65
Lewis, Oscar, 39
LGBTQ rights, 82
listening, as prayer, 178–80
Listening to Prozac (Kramer), 61, 68
literature, c/s/x movement
 becoming partners to c/s/x testimony, 115–19
 coercive psychiatry, 108–12
 consumer movement, 95–100
 ex-patients, structural factors, and need for narration, 100–2
 hearing voices, 102–8

literature, c/s/x movement—*Continued*
    mad liberation, 87–90
    On Our Own (Chamberlain), 83–6
    overview, 81–3
    social class and psychiatry, 112–15
    survivor movement and language of rights, 90–5
    themes and controversies in c/s/x movement, 86–7
    see also c/s/x movement

macro-social arrangements, 130, 164, 201
Madness News Network (MNN), 87–8, 117
Mahler, Jay, 87
Marxism, 31, 35, 65, 67, 83, 114–15, 156, 174
    see also Neo-Marxism
Medicaid, 6, 74
mental distress, social class and, 3–5
Mental Health Consumers' Self-Help Clearinghouse, 98
    see also self-help
meritocracy, 38, 134
methodological individualism, 5, 9, 63, 68, 77, 79, 106–7, 119, 164
Metzl, Jonathan, 69, 73
Meyer, Adolf, 65
micro-social arrangements, 130–1, 201
MindFreedom International, 92–4, 218n41
Minkowitz, Tina, 109
Moffatt, Ken, 143, 204n18
Morrison, Linda, 86, 89, 91–2
Moyers, Bill, 19
Muntaner, Carles, 32, 36, 42
Myrdal, Gunnar, 40
mysticism, 166–8
Myth of Mental Illness, The (Szasz), 66

National Alliance for the Mentally Ill (NAMI), 96, 98, 158

National Institute of Mental Health (NIMH), 69
neoliberalism
    alternatives to, 193–4
    capitalism and, 41, 43–4, 68, 156, 174
    consumer movement and, 95–6, 98–100
    counter-conducts and, 194–6
    defined, 3
    deinstitutionalization and, 75
    depression and, 64
    disability and, 37
    eschatology and, 174
    mental illness and, 36–7, 64, 78–9, 169
    mysticism and, 167
    pastoral counseling and, 14, 126–7, 129, 156–7
    pastoral theology interpreting, 44–7
    poverty and, 6, 40–1, 113–14, 138
    psychiatry and, 8–10, 80, 107
    psy-complex and, 7
    rights and, 183
    self-definition and, 112
    shame and, 126, 137, 184–5
    social class and, 3–5, 20, 23, 25, 28–31, 130, 166
    transinstitutionalization and, 82
    Wright on, 31–2, 34
Neo-Marxism, 31–2, 34, 36–7, 43
    see also Marxism
New England Journal of Medicine, 62
Nickel and Dimed (Ehrenreich), 135, 175
No Color Is My Kind (Cole), 199

Oaks, David, 87
Oates, Wayne, 178
O'Connor, Alice, 39
O'Connor v. Donaldson (1975), 108
Omnes et Singulatum, 159–60, 162
On Our Own (Chamberlin), 83

Packard, Elizabeth Parsons Ware, 69
Pastoral Care and Liberation Theology (Pattison), 76
pastoral counseling
　advocacy and group work, 143–9
　as interpretive, 126–9
　overview, 121–6, 153–4
　psy-complex and, 140–3
　recovering social teaching for, 149–52
　shame of poverty and, 134–5
　shame-affect bind and, 135–40
　social-class inquiry and, 129–34
pastoral power
　asceticism and, 171–2
　community and, 168–71
　counter-conducts of, 165–76
　eschatology and, 174–6
　explained, 159–62
　ministry and, 177–80
　monitoring mental illness, 157–9
　mysticism and, 166–7
　overview, 14–15, 155–7
　Scripture and, 172–4
　sources of, 162–5
Pattison, Stephen, 76
peer support, 13, 82–3, 85, 95, 107
penal system, 13, 145
　see also prisons
Perrucci, Robert, 49
Plato, 159
Pope Francis, 149
Pope Leo XIII, 149
Popper, Karl, 67
poverty
　CFT and, 144
　children and, 38–9
　c/s/x activism and, 105–6, 112–13, 144–5
　depression and, 21
　disability and, 36
　environment and, 27
　ethnicity and, 71, 127
　globalization and, 30

mental illness and, 30, 70, 76, 78, 99, 102, 105–7
ministry and, 47–8, 50
neoliberalism and, 6, 40–1, 113–14, 138
pastoral counseling and, 134–5, 148–9
psychology and, 123
psy-complex and, 7
shame and, 7, 16, 20, 39, 46, 122, 134–8, 153–4, 173
social class and, 9, 20, 38–44, 124–5
studies of, 27, 65
see also social class
prayer, 15, 166, 173, 176, 178–81, 183, 190, 193–4, 202
preferential option, 81, 181
Presence of God in Pastoral Counseling (Oates), 178
prisons, 16, 31, 41, 73–4, 82, 110, 201
Program for Assertive Community Treatment (PACT), 99, 108
Protest Psychosis, The (Metzl), 69
psychiatric advanced directives (PADs), 111–12
psychiatric diagnosis
　blaming the victim, 57–9
　conceptualizing suffering, 77–80
　deinstitutionalization and, managed care, 73–7
　discourse as productive truth, 55–7
　gender and race in, 69–73
　overview, 53–5
　pharmacology, 60–3
　return of descriptive psychiatry, 63–5
　rise of biomedical diagnostic psychiatry, 59–60
　social psychiatry and psychiatric auto-critique, 65–9
psychology
　marginalization of, 7–11
Psychology Today, 90

psy-complex
  biomedical model and, 15–16
  explained, 5–7
  identity and, 153
  methodological individualism and, 79
  ministry and, 164, 180
  pastoral counseling and, 124, 140–3
  poverty and, 7
  psychology and, 7–9, 72
  "public feeling," 4, 8, 160

racism, 9, 21, 36, 39–40, 65–6, 72, 78, 84, 92, 104, 107, 119, 137, 184
Raphael, Steven, 74
Rauschenbusch, Walter, 149
Reaching Out About Depression (ROAD), 144–5
Reagan, Ronald, 30, 39, 69, 74
research bias, 62
Resurrecting the Person (Swinton), 169
Reville, David, 112
Rieger, Joerg, 43, 49, 125, 134, 149–50, 172
Rogers, Joseph, 87, 98
Rogers v. Okin (1982), 108–9
Rogers-Vaughn, Bruce, 4, 9, 48, 64, 136, 204n14
Rojano, Ramón, 144
Rose, Lucy, 173
Rose, Nikolas, 5
Rosenhan, David L., 53–7, 91
Russell, Letty, 173
Ryan, John A., 150

sacrifice zones, 27
Saddleback Church, 157–8
  see also Warren, Rick
Sane Society, The (Fromm), 67
Santiago-Irizarry, Vilma, 70–1
Satel, Sally, 90
schizophrenia, 22, 53–4, 59, 63, 69–70, 72–4, 89–90, 100–2, 105–7, 115, 119, 192, 195

Scripture, 172–4
self-definition
  authority and, 89
  coercive psychiatry and, 108
  c/s/x activism and, 81, 83, 89, 107
  dignity and, 116
  explained, 81
  ministry and, 119
  neoliberalism and, 4
  pastoral counseling and, 119, 126
  self-determination and, 112, 185
  self-recovery and, 86
  social class and, 112, 115
  survivorship and, 92, 95
self-determination
  consumers and, 99
  c/s/x activism and, 13, 17, 81–2, 85–7, 89, 107
  disability and, 93
  explained, 81
  legal issues and, 109
  pastoral counseling and, 119
  self-definition and, 112, 115, 185
  social class and, 112
  survivorship and, 92
self-harm, 112, 115–17
self-help
  books, 75
  groups, 84, 88, 95
self-recovery movements, 86
Sen, Amartya, 136
sexism, 36, 70, 72, 78, 84, 92, 166
shame
  addressing, 122
  mental illness and, 94–5, 98, 191
  mysticism and, 168
  neoliberalism and, 126, 137, 184–5
  pastoral counseling and, 134–5, 160, 168, 198
  poverty, 7, 16, 20, 39, 46, 122, 134–8, 153–4, 173
  psychology and, 10
  shame-affect bind, 135–40

Index • 253

social class and, 122–3, 134–41, 151, 187
voicing experiences and, 8–9
shock treatments (ECT), 16, 88, 90, 92–4, 111, 118, 167
Slorach, Roddy, 114–15
Smail, David, 8
social class
　characteristics and traits for the poor, 37–41
　collective responsibility, 41–4
　desire, interest, and the excluded, 35–7
　economic conditions and mental illness, 21–6
　Erik Olin Wright's class analysis, 31–5
　ministry and, 47–9
　neoliberalism and, 3–5, 20, 23, 25, 28–31
　overview, 19–21, 49–51
　pastoral theology and, 44–7
　poverty and, 9, 20, 38–44
　stress, trauma, and causation, 27–8
Social Gospel, 126, 149–50, 152
Social Service Employee's Union, 87
Speaking Our Minds series, 105
St. Paul, 187–90
Stanley family, 19, 21–2, 44–5, 49–51
　see also *Two American Families*
Statsny, Peter, 111
Stearns, Eldrewery, 199–201
Stoll, Michael A., 74
suffering, conceptualizing, 77–80
suicide
　debt and, 25
　increase in rate of, 57, 67
　pharmaceuticals and, 62
　self-harm and, 115–16
　shame and, 136
　social class and, 3, 23–6
　stress and, 26
　unemployment and, 3, 23–4
Sullivan, Harry Stack, 9, 65

Sung, Jung Mo, 44
superstes, 116
suppression of research, 62
Survival and Liberation (Watkins-Ali), 127
survivors
　activism and, 96, 98, 112–14, 119
　chronicity and, 94–5
　consumerism and, 99
　disability and, 93
　explained, 13, 82
　hearing voices and, 103–4
　identity and, 89, 92, 95–7
　language and, 89–95
　mental health services and, 82
　mental illness and, 103–4
　methodological individualism and, 107
　ministry and, 119
　MNN and, 87
　narratives, 91, 166–7, 197–8
　partnership and, 115–17
　self-harm and, 115
　see also c/s/x movement
Swinton, John, 93, 168–9
Szasz, Thomas, 66–8, 87

Talking Back to Psychiatry (Morrison), 86
Tännsjö, Torbjörn, 109–11
testis, 116
Thandeka, 137
Topor, Alain, 100–2
Tran, Jonathan, 171
transinstitutionalization, 16, 82, 95
　see also deinstitutionalization; institutionalization
tricyclic drugs, 62
Two American Families (film), 19, 44
　see also Newman family; Stanley family

unemployment
　exclusion and, 35, 37
　gender/race and, 21, 72

unemployment—*Continued*
 globalization and, 68
 Great Recession and, 23–4, 26
 mental illness and, 3, 12, 15, 23–4, 59, 191
 ministry and, 45–6, 128, 172, 183
 prejudice and, 21
 recovery and, 101–2
 social class and, 1–2, 10
Untener, Ken, 202
Urantia, 178

Vietnam War, 74

Walker, Carl, 27, 30
Walker, Robert, 135–9

War against the Poor (Gans), 40
Warren, Rick, 157–8, 161
 see also Saddleback Church
Watkins-Ali, Carroll, 127, 143
Where We Stand (hooks), 8
Williams, Caesar, 70
Women and Madness (Chesler), 87
World Health Organization (WHO), 101–2
Wright, Erik Olin, 16, 31–5, 44, 49
Wysong, Earl, 49

Yan, Ming, 137

Zinman, Sally, 87

The manufacturer's authorised representative in the EU is Springer Nature Customer Service Centre GmbH, Europaplatz 3, 69115 Heidelberg, Germany. If you have any concerns regarding our products, please contact ProductSafety@springernature.com

Printed and bound by CPI Group (UK) Ltd, Croydon, CR0 4YY
23/03/2026
02076449-0018